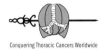

Conquering Thoracic Cancers Worldwide

SECOND EDITION

Staging Handbook in Thoracic Oncology

SECOND EDITION

Staging Handbook in Thoracic Oncology

Ramón Rami-Porta, MD, Executive Editor

An International Association for the Study of Lung Cancer Publication

Editorial Rx Press

North Fort Myers, FL

International Association for the Study of Lung Cancer
Aurora, CO, USA

Executive Editor: Ramón Rami-Porta, MD
Chair, IASLC Staging and Prognostic Factors Committee
Hospital Universitari Mútua Terrassa, University of Barcelona, Terrassa, Spain

An IASLC publication published by Editorial Rx Press

Editorial Rx Press, Registered Office: North Fort Myers, FL 33917
www.editorialrxpress.com

First Editorial Rx Press Printing 2016

10 9 8 7 6 5 4 3 2 1

ISBN: 978-0-9832958-6-0

Cover and interior design by Amy Boches, Biographics.
Use of the AJCC and UICC logos provided.

Dedication

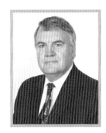

To Prof. Peter Goldstraw, MBChB, FRCS

Emeritus Professor of Thoracic Surgery,
National Heart and Lung Institute, Imperial College,

Honorary Consultant in Thoracic Surgery, Royal Brompton Hospital, London,

President (2011-2013), International Association for the Study
of Lung Cancer (IASLC),

Chair (1998-2009) and Past Chair (2009-2016), IASLC Staging and
Prognostic Factors Committee

With gratitude, esteem, and respect

Acknowledgments

The International Association for the Study of Lung Cancer (IASLC) expresses its most sincere gratitude to all the investigators and their institutions around the world for their voluntary contribution to the IASLC, the International Mesothelioma Interest Group (IMIG), the International Thymic Malignancies Interest Group (ITMIG) and the Worldwide Esophageal Cancer Collaboration (WECC) staging projects. Without their collaboration and submission of their cases, the data-based revisions leading to the 8th edition of the TNM classifications of thoracic malignancies would have not been possible. The complete list of contributors is in Rami-Porta R (ed), *IASLC Staging Manual in Thoracic Oncology*, 2nd edition; Editorial Rx Press, North Fort Myers, FL; 2016.

"Nought may endure but mutability!"

—Percy B. Shelley

Contents

Contents

Contributors

Editorial Committee

Executive Editor
Ramón Rami-Porta

Associate Editors
Hisao Asamura
Frank C. Detterbeck
Peter Goldstraw
Thomas W. Rice
Valerie W. Rusch

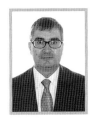

Ramón Rami-Porta

Members

Alex A. Adjei (Editor-in-Chief, Journal of Thoracic Oncology), Mayo Clinic, Rochester, MN, USA.

Hisao Asamura (Chair-Elect and Chair, N-Descriptors Subcommittee of the IASLC Staging and Prognostic Factors Committee, Japan Lung Cancer Society Liaison), Keio University, Tokyo, Japan.

Eugene H. Blackstone (Member of the Advisory Board of the IASLC Oesophageal Cancer Domain of the IASLC Staging and Prognostic Factors Committee, and the Worldwide Esophageal Cancer Collaboration), Cleveland Clinic, Cleveland, OH, USA.

James Brierley (Co-Chair, Union for International Cancer Control TNM Committee and UICC Liaison), Princess Margaret Cancer Centre/University Health Network, University of Toronto, Toronto, ON, Canada.

David Carbone (IASLC President), Ohio State's Comprehensive Cancer Center-James Cancer Hospital and Research Institute, Columbus, OH, USA.

John Crowley (Chief of Strategic Alliances), Cancer Research And Biostatistics, Seattle, WA, USA.

Frank C. Detterbeck (Chair, Thymic Malignancies Domain and Chair, Methodology and Validation Subcommittee of the IASLC Stating and Prognostic Factors Committee, and International Thymic Malignancies Interest Group Liaison), Yale University, New Haven, CT, USA.

Wilfried E. E. Eberhardt (Chair, M-Descriptors Subcommittee of the IASLC Staging and Prognostic Factors Committee), West German Cancer Centre, University Hospital, Ruhrlandklinik, Univesity Duisburg-Essen, Essen, Germany.

Pier Luigi Filosso (Member of the Advisory Board of the Thymic Malignancies Domain of the IASLC Staging and Prognostic Factors Committee), University of Torino, Torino, Italy.

Dorothy Giroux (Biostatistician), Cancer Research And Biostatistics, Seattle, WA, USA.

Peter Goldstraw (Past-President IASLC, Past-Chair IASLC Staging and Prognostic Factors Committee), Royal Brompton Hospital, Imperial College, London, UK.

Mary K. Gospodarowicz (Immediate Past President of the UICC, Co-Chair of the UICC TNM Core Group), Princess Margaret Hospital/University Health Network, University of Toronto, Toronto, Canada.

Fred R. Hirsch (CEO, IASLC and Board of Directors Liaison), University of Colorado Health Sciences, Denver, Colorado, USA.

Eng-Siew Koh, Princess Margaret Hospital/University Health Network, University of Toronto, Toronto, Canada.

Andrew G. Nicholson (Chair, Small Cell Lung Cancer Sub-committee of the IASLC Staging and Prognostic Factors Committee), Royal Brompton Hospital and Harefield NHS

Foundation Trust and Imperial College, London, UK.

Brian O'Sullivan (Chair, UICC Prognostic Factors Committee, Member of the UICC TNM Core Group), Princess Margaret Hospital/University Health Network, University of Toronto, Toronto, Canada.

Harvey I. Pass (Member of the Advisory Board of the IASLC Mesothelioma Domain of the IASLC Staging and Prognostic Factors Committee), New York University, New York, NY, USA.

Ramón Rami-Porta (Chair, IASLC Staging and Prognostic Factors Committee and Chair, Lung Cancer Domain and T-Descriptors Subcommittee), Hospital Universitari Mútua Terrassa, University of Barcelona, and Centros de Investigación Biomédica en Red de Enfermedades Respiratorias (CIBERES) Lung Cancer Group, Terrassa, Barcelona, Spain.

Thomas W. Rice (Chair, Carcinoma of the Oesophagus Domain of the IASLC Staging and Prognostic Factors Committee, and World Wide Esophageal Collaboration Liaison), Cleveland Clinic, Cleveland, OH, USA.

Valerie W. Rusch (Chair, Mesothelioma Domain of the IASLC Staging and Prognostic Factors Committee, and American Joint Committee on Cancer Liaison), Memorial Sloan-Kettering Cancer Center, New York, NY, USA.

Nagahiro Saijo (IASLC President 2007-2009), Former Deputy Director National Cancer Center East, Chiba, Executive Officer of the Japanese Society of Medical Oncology, Japan.

Jean-Paul Sculier (Chair, Prognostic Factors Subcommittee of the IASLC Staging and Prognostic Factors Committee), Institut Jules Bordet, Brussels, Belgium.

Lynn Shemanski (Senior Biostatistician), Cancer Research And Biostatistics, Seattle, WA, USA.

William D. Travis (Chair, Neuroendocrine Tumours Subcommittee of the IASLC Staging and Prognostic Factors Committee), Memorial Sloan-Kettering Cancer Center, New York, NY, USA.

Ming S. Tsao (Chair, Biologic Factors Subcommittee of the IASLC Staging and Prognostic Factors Committee), The Princess Margaret Cancer Centre, Toronto, Ontario, Canada.

The complete list of members of the IASLC Staging and Prognostic Factors Committee and of the Advisory Boards is in Rami-Porta R (ed), *IASLC Staging Manual in Thoracic Oncology*, 2nd edition; Editorial Rx Press, North Fort Myers, FL; 2016; and in the Appendix of the Introduction.

Preface to the Second Edition

By David P. Carbone, MD, PhD, IASLC President, 2015-2017,
and Fred R. Hirsch, MD, PhD, Chief Executive Officer

The staging of lung cancer and other thoracic malignancies is important for the treatment decisions. The Union for International Cancer Control/American Joint Committee on Cancer/International Association for the Study of Lung Cancer (UICC/AJCC/IASLC) Staging Classification is used all over the world and the IASLC is proud of launching the 8th Edition of the International Staging of Thoracic Malignancies. While the previous 7th Edition of the staging system was focusing on lung cancer, the new 8th Edition also includes staging of thymus cancers, malignant pleural mesothelioma, and carcinoma of the oesophagus. The new staging system is based on about 100.000 cases collected by international multidisciplinary investigators from all geographical regions of the world.

For the second consecutive time, the IASLC has been in charge to provide the UICC and the AJCC with data-based recommendations to revise the TNM classification of thoracic malignancies. Both institutions have accepted the IASLC recommendations and incorporated them in their respective 8th Edition staging manuals published in 2016.

The IASLC staging project has been performed by the IASLC Staging and Prognostic Factors Committee under the leadership of Dr. Ramón Rami-Porta, MD, Spain. This project could not be performed without the generous unrestricted support from Lilly Oncology, USA.

The IASLC is proud to serve the international oncological community and thanks the UICC and the AJCC for entrusting it with such challenging and intellectually rewarding responsibility. It is our hope that the 8th Edition of the Staging Classification will be a useful tool for further research and will serve in the daily lung cancer clinic to the benefit for the many patients with lung cancer around the world.

Introduction

By Ramón Rami-Porta, MD, PhD, FETCS, Executive Editor
Chair, IASLC Staging and Prognostic Factors Committee

The second phase of the International Association for the Study of Lung Cancer (IASLC) Staging Projects culminates with the publication of the second edition of the IASLC *Staging Manual in Thoracic Oncology* and the IASLC *Staging Handbook in Thoracic Oncology*. During these eight years since 2009, new datasets have been designed to register data on patients with lung cancer, malignant pleural mesothelioma and thymic tumours, and a memorandum of understanding was agreed with Dr. Thomas W. Rice, from the Cleveland Clinic, Cleveland, OH, USA, for an educational association to promote and disseminate the tumour, node and metastasis (TNM) classification of oesophageal cancer based on a new database of cases registered by the Worldwide Esophageal Cancer Collaboration (WECC). The IASLC also has worked in collaboration with the International Thymic Malignancies Interest Group (ITMIG) regarding the staging data of these tumours and with the International Mesothelioma Interest Group (IMIG), as well as with other organizations interested in the staging of malignant tumours, such as the European Society of Thoracic Surgeons, the Japanese Association for Research on the Thymus, and the Japanese Joint Committee for Lung Cancer Registry, among others. These entities and many institutions around the world sent data from their databases to Cancer Research And Biostatistics (CRAB) whose statisticians analysed and interpreted in close association with the members of the IASLC Staging and Prognostic Factors Committee and with the members of the newly created Advisory Boards. The Advisory

Boards consist of additional specialists who contribute their work and expertise to the IASLC Staging Projects. From the functional point of view, the members of the IASLC Staging and Prognostic Factors Committee were distributed in four different domains according to their areas of interest: Lung Cancer Domain, Malignant Pleural Mesothelioma Domain, Thymic Tumours Domain and Oesophageal Cancer Domain. (Appendix) Each domain has a chair, who is the link with the members of the Advisory Boards, and may have several sub-committees for specific tasks. (Figures 1 and 2)

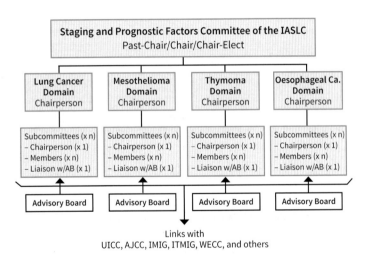

Figure 1. Structure of the International Association for the Study of Lung Cancer Staging and Prognostic Factors Committee. Notes: n: number; w: with; AB: Advisory Board; UICC: Union for International Cancer Control; AJCC: American Joint Committee on Cancer; IMIG: International Mesothelioma Interest Group; ITMIG: International Thymic Malignancies Interest Group; WECC: Worldwide Esophageal Cancer Collaboration.

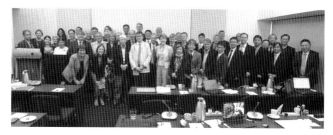

Figure 2. Most members of the International Association for the Study of Lung Cancer (IASLC) Staging and Prognostic Factors Committee met in Sydney, Australia, on October 25 and 26, 2013, prior to the 15th World Conference on Lung Cancer, to discuss the latest analyses of the IASLC database and decide on the recommendations for changes. This picture was taken at the end of the sessions on October 25, 2013.

The amount of collected data is huge. Table 1 shows the number of evaluable patients used for the revision of the TNM classifications of lung cancer, malignant pleural mesothelioma and oesophageal carcinoma, and for the development of an internationally agreed TNM classification for thymic malignancies. The analyses of the lung cancer database produced a series of original articles describing the characteristics of the database[1], the analyses, findings and

Table 1. Number of Evaluable Patients Used for Revision of the TNM Classifications of Thoracic Malignancies.

Tumour	Number of Evaluable Patients
Lung cancer*	77,156
Malignant pleural mesothelioma*	2,460
Thymic malignancies**	8,145
Oesophageal cancer***	22,654

* Registered by the International Association for the Study of Lung Cancer (IASLC) and analysed by Cancer Research And Biostatistics (CRAB).

** Registered by the International Thymic Malignancies Interest Group and the IASLC, and analysed by CRAB.

*** Registered by the World Wide Esophageal Cancer Collaboration and analysed at the Cleveland Clinic, Cleveland, OH, USA.

recommendations for changes on the T[2], the N[3], and the M[4] components of the classification, as well as those for the revision of the stages.[5] In addition, the recommended changes, based on the analyses of non-small cell lung cancer, were tested in the population of patients with small cell lung cancer. They were found to be useful in this cancer although the survival curves reflect the different natural history of small cell lung cancer and its worse prognosis.[6] The issue of how to classify lung cancers with multiple lesions was thoroughly discussed in four original papers on different patterns of disease: simultaneous second primaries,[7] separate tumour nodules,[8] multiple adenocarcinomas presenting as ground glass opacities on computed tomography and showing lepidic features on pathologic examination,[9] and adenocarcinoma with pneumonic pattern.[9] A succinct paper summarises the rules for classification and provides concise information on the criteria to classify these lesions at clinical and pathologic staging.[10] One additional article deals with the newly incorporated tumours into the TNM classification -adenocarcinoma *in situ* and minimally invasive adenocarcinoma- and how to code them in the 8th edition of the TNM classification of lung cancer.[11] Finally, another article discusses in detail the methodological aspects of the different analyses conducted for the 8th edition.[12]

Although more than a dozen classifications of thymic malignancies had been proposed during the past few decades, none was considered official or incorporated into the staging manuals of the American Joint Committee on Cancer and the Union for International Cancer Control. For the first time in the history of anatomic staging, a data-based, internationally and multidisciplinary agreed classification will be part of the 8th edition of the TNM classification of malignant tumours.

This thymic classification is, indeed, the first TNM-based internationally approved classification for this tumour site. The analyses of the IASLC/ITMIG database comprising more than 8,000 evaluable patients generated a series of original articles on the T[13] and the N and M components,[14] as well as on the stages[15] that have informed the proposed classification for the 8th edition staging manuals. A new lymph node map for exclusive use in thymic malignancies also has been proposed,[16] together with a revision of the mediastinal compartments.[17]

The analyses of the first IASLC mesothelioma database pointed out some limitations of the TNM classification.[18] Therefore, a call for the submission of more cases was launched resulting in the registration of 2,460 evaluable cases. Their analyses have generated four original articles, one on the database itself,[19] one on the T component,[20] another on the N component,[21] and another on the M component and stage grouping.[22] Not all limitations have been solved, but changes in the T and the N components, and in the stages have been suggested. In addition, an article on recommendations for uniform definitions of surgical procedures based on an IASLC/IMIG consensus was published,[23] as well as an article on prognostic factors.[24]

For the second consecutive time, the WECC database has been used to revise the TNM classification of oesophageal carcinoma. The initial one, used to inform the 7th edition of the classification, consisted of 4,627 patients who had undergone oesophageal resection with no induction therapy. Important innovations of this classification were the unification of the classification of oesophageal and oesophago-gastric junction cancers, and the introduction of non-anatomical parameters, such as cell type, histopathologic grade and tumour location, to arrange stage groupings. For the 8th edition, the WECC has data on 22,654 patients and, among these, there are patients whose tumours were clinically staged, pathologically staged and pathologically staged after induction therapy. The analyses of these three populations of patients have been reported in three articles that inform the 8th edition of the TNM classification of oesophageal cancer and oesophago-gastric junction.[25, 26, 27]

I would like to thank Prof. Peter Goldstraw, Past-Chair of the IASLC Staging and Prognostic Factors Committee. Far from retiring to an easy chair, he has actively participated in the development of all activities that have led to the 8th edition of the TNM classification of thoracic malignancies, sharing his knowledge, experience, common sense, diplomacy, political correctness and time, and contributing the most complex article in the series, i.e., the lung cancer stages article.[5] Ms. Deb Whippen, our publisher from Editorial Rx Press, already published the first edition of the IASLC *Staging Manual in Thoracic Oncology*[28] and the IASLC *Staging Handbook in Thoracic Oncology*,[29] has managed the production of their second edition. I thank her for her professionalism, enthusiasm, continuous availability and thoughtful suggestions. Dr. Aletta Anne Frazier, a radiologist by profession and a skillful medical illustrator, was kind enough to accept again our invitation to contribute her beautiful figures to the atlases of the different thoracic malignancies. I thank her for her dedication and good taste, and for devoting many hours of her time to the IASLC Staging Projects. It has been delightful to discuss with her over the phone the best options to illustrate the many categories of the four tumours included in the IASLC staging books. Nothing would have been possible without the data from our many contributors around the world. Their generosity is overwhelming. All are mentioned in the Acknowledgment section and I wholeheartedly thank them for their time, dedication and support. Ms. Dolores Martínez, Secretary to our Service of Thoracic Surgery, and Ms. Pat Vigues Frantzen, my Personal Assistant, have paid attention to every detail and have made my life much easier in so many ways that I cannot thank them enough. Finally, I would like to thank Dr. Fred Hirsch, IASLC CEO, IASLC presidents for this phase of the IASLC Staging Projects, Drs. David Gandara, Peter Goldstraw, Tony Mok and David Carbone, as well as all the IASLC Board Members, for their continuous support to the activities of the IASLC Staging and Prognostic Factors Committee.

As with the first edition, the second edition of the IASLC *Staging Manual in Thoracic Oncology* and the IASLC *Staging Handbook in Thoracic Oncology* has been produced in collaboration with the Union for International Cancer Control and the American Joint Committee on Cancer. Both institutions have granted us permission to reprint key chapters from their own books, which ensures uniformity in the three manuals. Their cooperation is much appreciated.

The IASLC Staging Projects, conceived in 1996 in London, during the International Workshop on Intrathoracic Staging, under the leadership of Prof. Peter Goldstraw and the sponsorship of the IASLC,[30] have already spanned for 20 years. After these two decades of continuous hard work, it is clear that the era of data-based revisions of the TNM classification of thoracic malignancies is consolidated. The work is not finished, though. The challenge of the combination of anatomic elements and non-anatomic elements, especially molecular markers, to construct prognostic groups and improve individualized prognosis will be the core activity of the third phase of the IASLC Staging Projects 2017-2024 that will be led by Dr. Hisao Asamura as Chair of the IASLC Staging and Prognostic

Factors Committee. We count, once more, on the data sent by our colleagues around the world to make this third phase, leading to the 9th edition of the TNM classification of thoracic malignancies, a scientific success and a useful contribution to our patients.

References

1. Rami-Porta R, Bolejack V, Giroux DJ et al. The IASLC Lung Cancer Staging Project: the new database to inform the eighth edition of the TNM classification of lung cancer. *J Thorac Oncol* 2014; 9: 1618-1624.

2. Rami-Porta R, Bolejack V, Crowley J et al. The IASLC Lung Cancer Staging Project: proposals for the revisions of the T descriptors in the forthcoming 8th edition of the TNM classification for lung cancer. *J Thorac Oncol* 2015; 10: 990-1003.

3. Asamura H, Chansky K, Crowley J et al. The IASLC Lung Cancer Staging Project: proposals for the revisions of the N descriptors in the forthcoming 8th edition of the TNM classification for lung cancer. *J Thorac Oncol* 2015; 10: 1675-1684.

4. Eberhardt WEE, Mitchell A, Crowley J et al. The IASLC Lung Cancer Staging Project: proposals for the revisions of the M descriptors in the forthcoming 8th edition of the TNM classification for lung cancer. *J Thorac Oncol* 2015; 10: 1515-1522.

5. Goldstraw P, Chansky K, Crowley J et al. The IASLC Lung Cancer Staging Project: proposals for the revision of the stage grouping in the forthcoming (8th) edition of the TNM classification of lung cancer. *J Thorac Oncol* 2016; 11: 39-51.

6. Nicholson AG, Chansky K, Crowley J et al. The IASLC Lung Cancer Staging Project: proposals for the revision of the clinical and pathologic staging of small cell lung cancer in the forthcoming eighth edition of the TNM classification for lung cancer. *J Thorac Oncol* 2016; 11: 300-311.

7. Detterbeck FC, Franklin WA, Nicholson AG et al. The IASLC Lung Cancer Staging Project: proposed criteria to distinguish separate primary lung cancers from metastatic foci in patients with two lung tumors in the forthcoming eighth edition of the TNM classification for lung cancer. *J Thorac Oncol* 2016; 11: 651-665.

8. Detterbeck FC, Bolejack V, Arenberg DA et al. The IASLC Lung Cancer Staging Project: proposals for the classification of lung cancer with

separate tumor nodules in the forthcoming eighth edition of the TNM classification for lung cancer. *J Thorac Oncol* 2016; 11: 681-692.

9. Detterbeck FC, Marom EM, Arenberg DA et al. The IASLC Lung Cancer Staging Project: proposals for the application of TNM staging rules to lung cancer presenting as multiple nodules with ground glass or lepidic features or a pneumonic-type of involvement in the forthcoming eighth edition of the TNM classification. *J Thorac Oncol* 2016; 11: 666-680.

10. Detterbeck FC, Nicholson AG, Franklin WA et al. The IASLC Lung Cancer Staging Project: proposals for revisions of the classification of lung cancers with multiple pulmonary sites of involvement in the forthcoming eighth edition of the TNM classification. *J Thorac Oncol* 2016; 11: 639-650.

11. Travis WD, Asamura H, Bankier A et al. The IASLC Lung Cancer Staging Project: proposals for coding T categories for subsolid nodules and assessment of tumor size in part-solid tumors in the forthcoming eighth edition of the TNM classification of lung cancer. *J Thorac Oncol* 2016; 11: 1204-1223.

12. Detterbeck F, Groome P, Bolejack V et al. The IASLC Lung Cancer Staging Project: methodology and validation used in the development of proposals for revision of the stage classification of non-small cell lung cancer in the forthcoming (eighth) edition of the TNM classification of lung cancer. *J Thorac Oncol* 2016; 11: 1433-1446.

13. Nicholson AG, Detterbeck FC, Marino M et al. The IASLC/ITMIG Thymic Epithelial Tumors Staging Project: proposals for the T component for the forthcoming (8th) edition of the TNM classification of malignant tumors. *J Thorac Oncol* 2014; 9 (suppl 2); s73-s80.

14. Kondo K, Van Schil P, Detterbeck FC at al. The IASLC/ITMIG Thymic Epithelial Tumors Staging Project: proposals for the N and M components for the forthcoming (8th) edition of the TNM classification of malignant tumors. *J Thorac Oncol* 2014; 9 (suppl 2): s81-s87.

15. Detterbeck FC, Stratton K, Giroux D et al. The IASLC/ITMIG Thymic Epithelial Tumors Staging Project: proposals for an evidence-based stage classification system for the forthcoming (8th) edition of the TNM classification of malignant tumors. *J Thorac Oncol* 2014; 9 (suppl 2): s65-s72.

16. Bhora FY, Chen DJ, Detterbeck FC et al. The ITMIG/IASLC Thymic Epithelial Tumors Staging Project: a proposed lymph node map for thymic epithelial tumors in the forthcoming 8th edition of the TNM classification of malignant tumors. *J Thorac Oncol* 2014; 9 (suppl 2): s88-s96.

17. Carter BW, Tomiyama N, Bhora FY et al. A modern definition of mediastinal compartments. *J Thorac Oncol* 2014; 9 (suppl 2): s97-s101.

18. Rusch VW, Giroux D, Kennedy C et al. Initial analysis of the International Association for the Study of Lung Cancer Mesothelioma database. *J Thorac Oncol* 2012; 7: 1631-1639.

19. Pass H, Giroux D, Kennedy C et al. The IASLC Mesothelioma database: improving staging of a rare disease through international participation. *J Thorac Oncol* 2016; in press.

20. Nowak AK, Chansky K, Rice DC et al. The IASLC Mesothelioma Staging Project: proposals for revisions of the T descriptors in the forthcoming eighth edition of the TNM classification for mesothelioma. *J Thorac Oncol* 2016; in press.

21. Rice D, Chansky K, Nowak A et al. The IASLC Mesothelioma Staging Project: proposals for revisions of the N descriptors in the forthcoming eighth edition of the TNM classification for malignant pleural mesothelioma. *J Thorac Oncol* 2016; in press.

22. Rusch VW, Chansky K, Kindler HL et al. The IASLC Malignant Pleural Mesothelioma Staging Project: proposals for the M descriptors and for the revision of the TNM stage groupings in the forthcoming (eighth) edition of the TNM classification for mesothelioma. *J Thorac Oncol* 2016; in press.

23. Rice D, Rusch V, Pass H et al. Recommendations for uniform definitions of surgical techniques for malignant pleural mesothelioma: a consensus report of the International Association for the Study of Lung Cancer International Staging Committee and the International Mesothelioma Interest Group. *J Thorac Oncol* 2011; 6: 1304-1312.

24. Pass HI, Giroux D, Kennedy C et al. Supplementary prognostic variables for pleural mesothelioma: a report from the IASLC Staging Committee. *J Thorac Oncol* 2014; 9: 856-864.

25. Rice TW, Apperson-Hansen C, DiPaola C et al. Worldwide Esophageal Cancer Collaboration: clinical staging data. *Dis Esophagus* 2016; 7: 707-714.

26. Rice TW, Chen L-Q, Hofstetter WL et al. Worldwide Esophageal Cancer Collaboration: pathologic staging data. *Dis Esophagus* 2016; 7: 724-733.

27. Rice TW, Lerut TEMR, Orringer MB et al. Worldwide Esophageal Cancer Collaboration: neoadjuvant pathologic staging data. *Dis Esophagus* 2016; 7: 715-723.

28. Goldstraw P, ed. IASLC *Staging Manual in Thoracic Oncology*. Editorial Rx Press, Orange, FL, USA; 2009.

29. Goldstraw P, ed. IASLC *Staging Handbook in Thoracic Oncology*. Editorial Rx Press, Orange, FL, USA; 2009.

30. Goldstraw P. Report on the international workshop on intrathoracic staging. London, October 1996. *Lung Cancer* 1997; 18: 107-111.

Appendix. Members and Structure of the IASLC Staging and Prognostic Factors Committee

Past-chair: Peter Goldstraw
Chair: Ramón Rami-Porta
Chair-elect: Hisao Asamura

LUNG CANCER DOMAIN
Chair: Ramón Rami-Porta

T Descriptors Subcommittee:
Ramón Rami-Porta (chair), David Ball, Vanessa Bolejack, John Crowley, Dorothy J. Giroux, Jhingook Kim, Gustavo Lyons, Thomas Rice, Kenji Suzuki, Charles F. Thomas Jr, William D. Travis, Yi-Iong Wu

N Descriptors Subcommittee:
Hisao Asamura (chair), David Ball, Kari Chansky, John Crowley, Peter Goldstraw, Valerie Rusch, Paul Van Schil, Johan Vansteenkiste, Hirokazu Watanabe, Yi-Iong Wu, Marcin Zielinski

M Descriptors Subcommittee:
Wilfried Eberhardt (chair), Kari Chansky, John Crowley, Young Tae Kim, Haruhiko Kondo, Alan Mitchell, Andrew Turrisi

Validation and Methodology Subcommittee:
Patti Groome (chair 2010-15), Frank Detterbeck (chair 2015-7), Vanessa Bolejack, John Crowley, Catherine Kennedy, Mark Krasnik, Michael Peak

Prognostic Factors Subcommittee:
Jean-Paul Sculier (chair), Kari Chansky, John Crowley, Dorothy J. Giroux, Fergus Gleeson, Jan van Meeerbeeck

Neuroendocrine Tumours Subcommittee:
William D. Travis (chair), Hisao Asamura, Kari Chansky, John Crowley, Dorothy J. Giroux

Small Cell Lung Cancer Subcommittee:
Andrew Nicholson (chair), Ricardo Beyruti, Kari Chansky, John Crowley, Kouru Kubota, Andrew Turrisi

Biologic Factors Subcommittee:
Ming S. Tsao (chair), David G. Beer, John Crowley, Yi-Iong Wu

T Coding and Size Measurement in Preinvasive and Lepidic Adenocarcinoma ad hoc *Workgroup:*
William D. Travis (chair), Hisao Asamura, Alex Bankier, Mary Beth Beasley, Frank Detterbeck, Douglas B. Flieder, Jin Mo Goo, Heber MacMahon, David Naidich, Andrew Nicholson, Charles A. Powell, Mathias Prokop, Ramón Rami-Porta, Valerie Rusch, Paul Van Schil, Yasushi Yatabe

Multiple Pulmonary Sites of Involvement ad hoc *Workgroup:*
Frank Detterbeck (chair), Douglas A. Arenberg, Hisao Asamura, Vanessa Bolejack, John Crowley, Jessica S. Donington, Wilbur A. Franklin, Nicolas Girard, Edith M. Marom, Peter J. Mazzone, Andrew G. Nicholson, Valerie W. Rusch, Lynn T. Tanoue, William D. Travis

MALIGNANT PLEURAL MESOTHELIOMA DOMAIN
Chair: Valerie Rusch
Hisao Asamura, John Crowley, John G. Edwards, Françoise Galateau-Sallé, Dorothy J. Giroux, Catherine Kennedy, Jan van Meerbeeck, Takashi Nakano, Anna Nowack, K. E. Rosenzweig, William Travis, Johan Vansteenkiste

Mesothelioma Advisory Board:
Liaison with the Malignant Pleural Mesothelioma Domain: Valerie Rusch
Members: Paul Baas, Seiki Hasegawa, Jeremy Erasmus, Kouki Inai, Kemp Kernstein, Hedy Kindler, Lee Krug, Kristiaan Nackaerts, Harvey Pass, David Rice

THYMIC MALIGNANCIES DOMAIN
Chair: Frank Detterbeck
Hisao Asamura, John Crowley, Dorothy Giroux, James Huang, Jhingook Kim, Mirella Marino, Edith Marom, Anderew Nicholson, Enrico Ruffini, Paul Van Schil

Thymic Malignancies Advisory Board:
Liaison with the Thymic Malignancies Domain: Frank Detterbeck
Members: Conrad Falkson, Pier Luigi Filosso, Giuseppe Giaccone, Kazuya Kondo, Mario Lucchi, Meinoshin Okumura

OESOPHAGEAL CARCINOMA DOMAIN
Chair: Thomas Rice
John Crowley, Toni Lerut, Yuji Tachimori

Oesophageal Carcinoma Advisory Board:
Liaison with the Oesophageal Carcinoma Domain: Thomas Rice
Member: Eugene Blackstone

PART I

GENERAL

Acknowledgment: Used with the permission of the Union for International Cancer Control (UICC), Geneva, Switzerland. The original source for this material is in Brierley JB, Gospodarowicz MK, Wittekind C, eds. UICC TNM Classification of Malignant Tumours, 8th edition (2017), published by John Wiley & Sons, Ltd, www.wiley.com.

1

The Principles of the TNM System

The practice of classifying cancer cases into groups according to anatomical extent, termed 'stage', arose from the observation that survival rates were higher for cases in which the disease was localized than for those in which the disease had extended beyond the organ of origin. The stage of disease at the time of diagnosis is a reflection not only of the rate of growth and extension of the neoplasm but also the type of tumour and the tumour–host relationship.

It is important to record accurate information on the anatomical extent of the disease for each site at the time of diagnosis, to meet the following objectives:

1. to aid the clinician in the planning of treatment
2. to give some indication of prognosis for survival
3. to assist in evaluation of the results of treatment
4. to facilitate the exchange of information between treatment centres
5. to contribute to the continuing investigation of human cancer
6. to support cancer control activities.

Cancer staging is essential to patient care, research, and cancer control. Cancer control activities include direct patient care-related activities, the development and implementation of clinical practice guidelines, and centralized activities such as recording disease extent in cancer registries for surveillance purposes and planning cancer systems. Recording of stage is essential for the evaluation of outcomes of clinical practice and cancer programmes. However, in order to evaluate the long-term outcomes of populations, it is important for the classification to remain stable. There is therefore a conflict between a classification that is updated to include the most current forms of medical knowledge while also maintaining a classification that facilitates longitudinal studies. The UICC TNM Project aims to address both needs.

International agreement on the classification of cancer by extent of disease provides a method of conveying disease extent to others without ambiguity.

There are many axes of tumour classification: for example, the anatomical site and the clinical and pathological extent of disease, the duration of symptoms or signs, the gender and age of the patient, and the histological type and grade of the tumour. All of these have an influence on the outcome of the disease. Classification by anatomical extent of disease is the one with which the TNM system primarily deals.

The clinician's immediate task when meeting a patient with a new diagnosis of cancer is to make a judgment as to prognosis and a decision as to the most effective course of treatment. This judgment and this decision require, among other things, an objective assessment of the anatomical extent of the disease.

To meet the stated objectives a system of classification is needed:

1. that is applicable to all sites regardless of treatment; and
2. that may be supplemented later by further informa-

tion that becomes available from histopathology and/or surgery.

The TNM system meets these requirements.

The General Rules of the TNM System[a,b]

The TNM system for describing the anatomical extent of disease is based on the assessment of three components:

 T – the extent of the primary tumour

 N – the absence or presence and extent of regional lymph node metastasis

 M – the absence or presence of distant metastasis.

The addition of numbers to these three components indicates the extent of the malignant disease, thus:

 T0, T1, T2, T3, T4, N0, N1, N2, N3, M0, M1

In effect, the system is a 'shorthand notation' for describing the extent of a particular malignant tumour.

The general rules applicable to all sites are as follows:

1. All cases should be confirmed microscopically. Any cases not so proved must be reported separately.

2. Two classifications are described for each site, namely:

   a) **Clinical classification:** the pretreatment clinical classification designated **TNM** (or cTNM) is essential to select and evaluate therapy. This is based on evidence acquired before treatment. Such evidence is gathered from physical examination, imaging, endoscopy, biopsy, surgical exploration, and other relevant examinations.

   b) **Pathological classification:** the postsurgical histopathological classification, designated **pTNM**, is used to guide adjuvant therapy and provides additional data to estimate prognosis and end results. This is based on evidence acquired before treatment, supplemented or modified by additional evidence acquired from surgery and from pathological examination. The pathological assessment of the primary tumour (pT) entails a resection of the primary tumour or biopsy adequate to evaluate the highest pT category. The pathological assessment of the regional lymph nodes (pN) entails removal of the lymph nodes adequate to validate the absence of regional lymph node metastasis (pN0) or sufficient to evaluate the highest pN category. An excisional biopsy of a lymph node without pathological assessment of the primary is insufficient to fully evaluate the pN category and is a clinical classification. The pathological assessment of distant metastasis (pM) entails microscopic examination of metastatic deposit.

3. After assigning T, N, and M and/or pT, pN, and pM categories, these may be grouped into stages.The TNM classification and stages, are established at diagnosis and must remain unchanged in the medical records. Only for cancer surveillance purposes, clinical and pathological data may be combined when only partial information is available either in the pathological classification or the clinical classification.

4. If there is doubt concerning the correct T, N, or M category to which a particular case should be allotted, then the lower (i.e., less advanced) category should be chosen. This will also be reflected in the stage.

5. In the case of multiple primary tumours in one organ, the tumour with the highest T category should be classified and the multiplicity or the number of tumours should be indicated in parenthesis, e.g., T2(m) or T2(5). In simultaneous bilateral primary cancers of paired organs, each

tumour should be classified independently. In tumours of the liver, ovary and fallopian tube, multiplicity is a criterion of T classification, and in tumours of the lung multiplicity may be a criterion of the M classification.

6. Definitions of the TNM categories and stage may be telescoped or expanded for clinical or research purposes as long as the basic definitions recommended are not changed. For instance, any T, N, or M can be divided into subgroups.

Notes

[a]For more details on classification the reader is referred to the TNM Supplement.

[b]An educational module is available on the UICC website www.uicc.org.

Anatomical Regions and Sites

The sites in this classification are listed by code number of the International Classification of Diseases for Oncology.[1] Each region or site is described under the following headings:

- Rules for classification with the procedures for assessing the T, N, and M categories
- Anatomical sites, and subsites if appropriate
- Definition of the regional lymph nodes
- TNM Clinical classification
- pTNM Pathological classification
- G Histopathological grading if different from that described in the Histopathological Grading section provided further in this chapter
- Stage and prognostic groups
- Prognostic factors grid

TNM Clinical Classification

The following general definitions are used throughout:

T – Primary Tumour

TX   Primary tumour cannot be assessed
T0   No evidence of primary tumour
Tis   Carcinoma in situ
T1–T4   Increasing size and/or local extent of the primary
        tumour

N – Regional Lymph Nodes

NX   Regional lymph nodes cannot be assessed
N0   No regional lymph node metastasis
N1–N3   Increasing involvement of regional lymph nodes

M – Distant Metastasis*

M0   No distant metastasis
M1   Distant metastasis

Note

*The MX category is considered to be inappropriate as clinical assessment of metastasis can be based on physical examination alone. (The use of MX may result in exclusion from staging.)

The category M1 may be further specified according to the following notation:

Pulmonary	PUL (C34)	Brain	BRA (C71)
Bone marrow	MAR (C42.1)	Adrenals	ADR (C74)
Osseous	OSS (C40, 41)	Lymph nodes	LYM (C77)
Pleura	PLE (C38.4)	Skin	SKI (C44)
Hepatic	HEP (C22)	Others	OTH
Peritoneum	PER (C48.1,2)		

Subdivisions of TNM

Subdivisions of some main categories are available for those who need greater specificity (e.g., T1a, T1b or N2a, N2b).

pTNM Pathological Classification

The following general definitions are used throughout:

pT – Primary Tumour

pTX   Primary tumour cannot be assessed histologically
pT0   No histological evidence of primary tumour
pTis   Carcinoma in situ
pT1–4   Increasing size and/or local extent of the primary tumour histologically

pN – Regional Lymph Nodes

pNX   Regional lymph nodes cannot be assessed histologically
pN0   No regional lymph node metastasis histologically
pN1–3   Increasing involvement of regional lymph nodes histologically

Notes

- Direct extension of the primary tumour into lymph nodes is classified as lymph node metastasis.
- Tumour deposits (satellites), i.e., macro- or microscopic nests or nodules, in the lymph drainage area of a primary carcinoma without histological evidence of residual lymph node in the nodule, may represent discontinuous spread, venous invasion (V1/2) or a totally replaced lymph node. If a nodule is considered by the pathologist to be a totally replaced lymph node (generally having a smooth contour), it should be recorded as a positive lymph node, and each such nodule should be counted separately as a lymph node in the final pN determination.

- Metastasis in any lymph node other than regional is classified as a distant metastasis.
- When size is a criterion for pN classification, measurement is made of the metastasis, not of the entire lymph node. The measurement should be that of the largest dimension of the tumour.
- Cases with micrometastasis only, i.e., no metastasis larger than 0.2 cm, can be identified by the addition of '(mi)', e.g., pN1(mi).

Sentinel Lymph Node

The sentinel lymph node is the first lymph node to receive lymphatic drainage from a primary tumour. If it contains metastatic tumour this indicates that other lymph nodes may contain tumour. If it does not contain metastatic tumour, other lymph nodes are not likely to contain tumour. Occasionally, there is more than one sentinel lymph node.

The following designations are applicable when sentinel lymph node assessment is attempted:

(p)NX(sn)   Sentinel lymph node could not be assessed
(p)N0(sn)   No sentinel lymph node metastasis
(p)N1(sn)   Sentinel lymph node metastasis

Isolated Tumour Cells

Isolated tumour cells (ITC) are single tumour cells or small clusters of cells not more than 0.2 mm in greatest extent that can be detected by routine H and E stains or immunohisto-chemistry. An additional criterion has been proposed in breast cancer to include a cluster of fewer than 200 cells in a single histological cross-section. Others have proposed for other tumour sites that a cluster should have 20 cells or fewer; definitions of ITC may vary by tumour site. ITCs do not typically show evidence of metastatic activity (e.g., proliferation or stromal reaction) or penetration of vascular or lymphatic sinus walls.

Cases with ITC in lymph nodes or at distant sites should be classified as N0 or M0, respectively. The same applies to cases with findings suggestive of tumour cells or their components by non-morphological techniques such as flow cytometry or DNA analysis. The exceptions are in malignant melanoma of the skin and Merkel cell carcinoma, wherein ITC in a lymph node are classified as N1. These cases should be analysed separately.[2] Their classification is as follows.

(p)N0	No regional lymph node metastasis histologically, no examination for isolated tumour cells (ITC)
(p)N0(i–)	No regional lymph node metastasis histologically, negative morphological findings for ITC
(p)N0(i+)	No regional lymph node metastasis histologically, positive morphological findings for ITC
(p)N0(mol–)	No regional lymph node metastasis histologically, negative non-morphological findings for ITC
(p)N0(mol+)	No regional lymph node metastasis histolog cally, positive non-morphological findings for ITC

Cases with or examined for isolated tumour cells (ITC) in sentinel lymph nodes can be classified as follows:

(p)N0(i–)(sn)	No sentinel lymph node metastasis histologically, negative morphological findings for ITC
(p)N0(i+)(sn)	No sentinel lymph node metastasis histologically, positive morphological findings for ITC
(p)N0(mol–)(sn)	No sentinel lymph node metastasis histologically, negative non-morphological findings for ITC

(p)N0 (mol+)(sn)   No sentinel lymph node metastasis histologically, positive non-morphological findings for ITC

pM – Distant Metastasis*
pM1   Distant metastasis microscopically confirmed

Note
*pM0 and pMX are not valid categories.

The category pM1 may be further specified in the same way as M1 (see TNM Clinical Classification section provided earlier in this chapter).

Isolated tumour cells found in bone marrow with morphological techniques are classified according to the scheme for N, e.g., M0(i+). For non-morphological findings 'mol' is used in addition to M0, e.g., M0 (mol+).

Histopathological Grading
In most sites, further information regarding the primary tumour may be recorded under the following heading:

G – Histopathological Grading
GX   Grade of differentiation cannot be assessed
G1   Well differentiated
G2   Moderately differentiated
G3   Poorly differentiated
G4   Undifferentiated

Notes
- Grades 3 and 4 can be combined in some circumstances as 'G3-4, poorly differentiated or undifferentiated'.

- Special systems of grading are recommended for tumours of breast, corpus uteri, and prostate.

Additional Descriptors

For identification of special cases in the TNM or pTNM classification, the m, y, r, and a symbols may be used. Although they do not affect the stage grouping, they indicate cases needing separate analysis.

m Symbol. The suffix m, in parentheses, is used to indicate the presence of multiple primary tumours at a single site. See TNM rule no. 5.

y Symbol. In those cases in which classification is performed during or following multimodality therapy, the cTNM or pTNM category is identified by a y prefix. The ycTNM or ypTNM categorizes the extent of tumour actually present at the time of that examination. The y categorization is not an estimate of the extent of tumour prior to multimodality therapy.

r Symbol. Recurrent tumours, when classified after a disease-free interval, are identified by the prefix r.

a Symbol. The prefix a indicates that classification is first determined at autopsy.

Optional Descriptors
L – Lymphatic Invasion

LX   Lymphatic invasion cannot be assessed
L0   No lymphatic invasion
L1   Lymphatic invasion

V – Venous Invasion

VX   Venous invasion cannot be assessed
V0   No venous invasion
V1   Microscopic venous invasion
V2   Macroscopic venous invasion

Note

Macroscopic involvement of the wall of veins (with no tumour within the veins) is classified as V2.

Pn – Perineural Invasion

PnX   Perineural invasion cannot be assessed
Pn0   No perineural invasion
Pn1   Perineural invasion

Residual Tumour (R) Classification*

The absence or presence of residual tumour after treatment is described by the symbol R. More details can be found in the TNM Supplement (see Preface, Reference 3).

TNM and pTNM describe the anatomical extent of cancer in general without considering treatment. They can be supplemented by the R classification, which deals with tumour status after treatment. It reflects the effects of therapy, influences further therapeutic procedures, and is a strong predictor of prognosis.

The definitions of the R categories are:

RX   Presence of residual tumour cannot be assessed
R0   No residual tumour
R1   Microscopic residual tumour
R2   Macroscopic residual tumour.

Note

*Some consider the R classification to apply only to the primary tumour and its local or regional extent. Others have applied it more broadly to include distant metastasis. The specific usage should be indicated when the R is used.

Stage and Prognostic Groups

The TNM system is used to describe and record the anatomical extent of disease. For purposes of tabulation and analysis it is useful to condense these categories into groups. For consistency, in the TNM system, carcinoma in situ is categorized stage 0; in general, tumours localized to the organ of origin as stages I and II, locally extensive spread, particularly to regional lymph nodes as stage III, and those with distant metastasis as stage IV. The stage adopted is such as to ensure, as far as possible, that each group is more or less homogeneous in respect of survival, and that the survival rates of these groups for each cancer site are distinctive.

For pathological stages, if sufficient tissue has been removed for pathological examination to evaluate the highest T and N categories, M1 may be either clinical (cM1) or pathological (pM1). However, if only a distant metastasis has had microscopic confirmation, the classification is pathological (pM1) and the stage is pathological.

Although the anatomical extent of disease, as categorized by TNM, is a very powerful prognostic indicator in cancer, it is recognized that many factors have a significant impact on predicting outcomes. This has resulted in different stage groups. In thyroid cancer there are different stage definitions for different histologies and, new to this edition, in oropharyngeal cancer HPV-related cancer is staged differently from non-HPV-related cancer. Some factors have been combined with TNM in the development of stage groupings; for instance, for different histologies (thyroid), different major prognostic factor groups (age in thyroid), and by aetiology (HPV-related oropharyngeal cancer). In this edition the term **stage** has been used as defining the anatomical extent of disease while **prognostic group** for classifications that incorporate other prognostic factors. Historically, age in differentiated thyroid cancer and grade in soft tissue sarcoma are combined with anatomical extent of disease to determine stage, and stage is retained rather than prognostic group in these two sites.

Prognostic Factors Classification

Prognostic factors can be classified as those pertaining to:

- **Anatomic extent of disease:** describes the extent of disease in the patient at the time of diagnosis. Classically, this is TNM but may also include tumour markers that reflect tumour burden, for instance prostate-specific antigen (PSA) in prostate carcinoma or carcinoembryonic antigen (CEA) in colorectal carcinoma.
- **Tumour profile:** this includes pathological (i.e., grade) and molecular features of a tumour, and gene expression patterns that reflect behaviour. These can be:
  - predictive factors
  - prognostic factors
  - companion diagnostic marker
- **Patient profile:** this includes terms related to the host of the cancer. These can be demographic factors, such as age and gender, or acquired, such as immunodeficiency and performance status.
- **Environment:** this may include treatment-related and education (expertise, access, ageism, and healthcare delivery) and quality of management.

When describing prognostic factors it is important to state what outcome the factors are prognostic for, and at what point in the patient trajectory. Anatomical extent of disease as described by TNM stage defines prognosis for survival.

In the second edition of the *UICC Prognostic Factors in Cancer* for each tumour site, grids were developed that identified prognostic factors for survival at time of diagnosis and whether they were considered to be essential, additional, or new and promising.[3] The grids were updated for the third edition[4] and have been further updated and incorporated into the ninth edition of the *UICC Manual of Clinical Oncology*.[5] Essential factors are those that are required in addition to anatomical extent of disease to determine treatment as identified by published clinical practice guidelines. The table is a generic example of the prognostic factors summary grid. The grids from the ninth edition of the *UICC Manual of Clinical Oncology* are reproduced in this eighth edition. Grids are not available for some of the less common tumours.

Examples of the UICC prognostic factors summary 'grid'

Prognostic Factors	Tumour Related	Host Related	Environment Related
Essential*	Anatomical disease extent Histological type	Age	Availability of access to radiotherapy
Additional	Tumour bulk Tumour marker level Programmed death 1 (PD-1) receptor and its ligands (PD-L1)	Race Gender Cardiac function	Expertise of a treatment at the specific level (e.g., surgery or radiotherapy)
New and promising	Epidermal growth factor receptor Gene expression patterns	Germline *p53*	Access to information

The origin of essential factors as imperatives for treatment decisions are from known and available clinical practice guidelines.

Essential TNM

Information on anatomical extent of disease at presentation or stage is central to cancer surveillance to determine cancer burden as it provides additional valuable information to incidence and mortality data.[6] However, cancer registries in low and middle income countries frequently have insufficient information to determine complete TNM data, either because of inability to perform necessary investigations or because of lack of recording of information. In view of this, the UICC TNM Project has with the International Agency for Research in Cancer and the National Cancer Institute developed a new classification system 'Essential TNM' that can be used to collect stage data when complete information is not available. To date, Essential TNM schemas have been developed for breast, cervix, colon, and prostate cancer, and are presented in this edition and available for download at www.uicc.org.

Paediatric Tumours

Since the fourth edition, the *UICC TNM Classification of Malignant Tumours* has not incorporated any classifications of paediatric tumours. This decision has stemmed from the lack of an international standard staging system for many paediatric tumours. To enable stage data collection by population-based cancer registries there needs to be agreement on cancer staging. Recognition of this led to a consensus meeting held in 2014 and resulted in the publication of recommendations on the staging of paediatric malignancies for the purposes of population surveillance.[7] The classifications published are not intended to replace the classifications used by the clinician when treating an individual patient but instead to facilitate the collection of stage by population-based cancer registries.

Related Classifications

Since 1958, WHO has been involved in a programme aimed at providing internationally acceptable criteria for the histological diagnosis of tumours. This has resulted in the *International Histological Classification of Tumours,* which contains, in an illustrated multivolume series, definitions of tumour types and a proposed nomenclature. A new series, *WHO Classification of Tumours–Pathology and Genetics of Tumours*, continues this effort. (Information on these publications is at www.iarc.fr).

The *WHO International Classification of Diseases for Oncology (ICD-O-3)*[1] is a coding system for neoplasms by topography and morphology and for indicating behaviour (e.g., malignant, benign). This coded nomenclature is identical in the morphology field for neoplasms to the Systematized Nomenclature of Medicine (SNOMED).[8]

In the interest of promoting national and international collaboration in cancer research and specifically of facilitating cooperation in clinical investigations, it is recommended that the WHO *Classification of Tumours* be used for classification and definition of tumour types and that the ICD-O-3 code be used for storage and retrieval of data.

References

1. Fritz A, Percy C, Jack A, Shanmugaratnam K, Sobin L, Parkin DM, Whelan S, eds. *WHO International Classification of Diseases for Oncology ICD-O*, 3rd edn. Geneva: WHO, 2000.
2. Hermanek P, Hutter RVP, Sobin LH, Wittekind Ch. Classification of isolated tumour cells and micrometastasis. *Cancer* 1999; 86: 2668–2673.
3. International Union Against Cancer (UICC) Gospodarowicz MK, Henson DE, Hutter RVP, et al., eds. *Prognostic Factors in Cancer*, 2nd edn. New York: Wiley, 2001.
4. International Union Against Cancer (UICC) Gospodarowicz MK, O'Sullivan B, Sobin LH, eds. *Prognostic Factors in Cancer*, 3rd edn. New York: Wiley, 2006.
5. O'Sullivan B, Brierley J, D'Cruz A, Fey M, Pollock R, Vermorken J, Huang S. *Manual of Clinical Oncology*, 9th edn. Oxford: Wiley-Blackwell, 2015.

6. The World Health Organization. *Cancer Control Knowledge into Action, Guide for Effective Programs*. Available at: www.who.int/cancer/modules/en/(accessed Aug. 2016).

7. Gupta S, Aitken J, Bartels U, et al. Paediatric cancer stage in population-based cancer registries: the Toronto consensus principles and guidelines. *Lancet Oncol* 2016; 17: e163–172.

8. SNOMED International: *The Systematized Nomenclature of Human and Veterinary Medicine*. Northfield, Ill: College of American Pathologists. Available at: www.cap.org (accessed Aug. 2016).

PART II

LUNG CANCER

Acknowledgment: Used with the permission of the Union for International Cancer Control (UICC), Geneva, Switzerland. The original source for this material is in Brierley JB, Gospodarowicz MK, Wittekind Ch, eds. UICC TNM Classification of Malignant Tumours, 8th edition (2017), published by John Wiley & Sons, Ltd, www.wiley.com.

2

8th Edition of TNM for Lung Cancer

Introductory Notes

The classification applies to carcinomas of the lung including non-small cell and small cell carcinomas, and bronchopulmonary carcinoid tumours.

Each site is described under the following headings:

- Rules for classification with the procedures for assessing T, N, and M categories; additional methods may be used when they enhance the accuracy of appraisal before treatment
- Anatomical subsites where appropriate
- Definition of the regional lymph nodes
- TNM clinical classification
- pTNM pathological classification
- Stage
- Prognostic factors grid

Regional Lymph Nodes

The regional lymph nodes extend from the supraclavicular region to the diaphragm. Direct extension of the primary tumour into lymph nodes is classified as lymph node metastasis.

Lung
(ICD-O-3 C34)
Rules for Classification

The classification applies to carcinomas of the lung including non-small cell carcinomas, small cell carcinomas, and bronchopulmonary carcinoid tumours. It does not apply to sarcomas and other rare tumours.

Changes in this edition from the seventh edition are based upon recommendations from the International Association for the Study of Lung Cancer (IASLC) Staging Project (see references).[1-6]

There should be histological confirmation of the disease and division of cases by histological type.

The following are the procedures for assessing T, N, and M categories:

T categories	Physical examination, imaging, endoscopy, and/or surgical exploration
N categories	Physical examination, imaging, endoscopy, and/or surgical exploration
M categories	Physical examination, imaging, and/or surgical exploration

Anatomical Subsites

1. Main bronchus (C34.0)
2. Upper lobe (C34.1)
3. Middle lobe (C34.2)
4. Lower lobe (C34.3)

Regional Lymph Nodes

The regional lymph nodes are the intrathoracic nodes (mediastinal, hilar, lobar, interlobar, segmental, and subsegmental), scalene, and supraclavicular lymph nodes.

TNM Clinical Classification
T – Primary Tumour

TX   Primary tumour cannot be assessed, or tumour proven by the presence of malignant cells in sputum or bronchial washings but not visualized by imaging or bronchoscopy

T0   No evidence of primary tumour

Tis Carcinoma *in situ*[a]

T1   Tumour 3 cm or less in greatest dimension, surrounded by lung or visceral pleura, without bronchoscopic evidence of invasion more proximal than the lobar bronchus (i.e., not in the main bronchus)[b]

  T1mi Minimally invasive adenocarcinoma[c]

  T1a   Tumour 1 cm or less in greatest dimension[b]

  T1b   Tumour more than 1 cm but not more than 2 cm in greatest dimension[b]

  T1c   Tumour more than 2 cm but not more than 3 cm in greatest dimension[b]

T2   Tumour more than 3 cm but not more than 5 cm; or tumour with *any* of the following features[d]

  • Involves main bronchus regardless of distance to the carina, but without involvement of the carina

  • Invades visceral pleura

  • Associated with atelectasis or obstructive pneumonitis that extends to thehilar region either involving part of or the entire lung

  T2a   Tumour more than 3 cm but not more than 4 cm in greatest dimension

  T2b   Tumour more than 4 cm but not more than 5 cm in greatest dimension

T3   Tumour more than 5 cm but not more than 7 cm in greatest dimension or one that directly invades any of the following: parietal pleura, chest wall (including superior sulcus tumours), phrenic nerve, parietal pericardium; or separate tumour nodule(s) in the same lobe as the primary

T4   Tumour more than 7 cm or of any size that invades any of the following: diaphragm, mediastinum, heart, great vessels, trachea, recurrent laryngeal nerve, oesophagus, vertebral body, carina; separate tumour nodule(s) in a different ipsilateral lobe to that of the primary

N – Regional Lymph Nodes

NX   Regional lymph nodes cannot be assessed

N0   No regional lymph node metastasis

N1   Metastasis in ipsilateral peribronchial and/or ipsilateral hilar lymph nodes and intrapulmonary nodes, including involvement by direct extension

N2   Metastasis in ipsilateral mediastinal and/or subcarinal lymph node(s)

N3   Metastasis in contralateral mediastinal, contralateral hilar, ipsilateral or contralateral scalene, or supraclavicular lymph node(s)

M – Distant Metastasis

M0   No distant metastasis

M1   Distant metastasis

M1a   Separate tumour nodule(s) in a contralateral lobe; tumour with pleural or pericardial nodules or malignant pleural or pericardial effusion[e]

M1b   Single extrathoracic metastasis in a single organ[f]

M1c   Multiple extrathoracic metastasis in a single or multiple organs

Notes

[a] Tis includes adenocarcinoma *in situ* and squamous carcinoma *in situ*.

[b] The uncommon superficial spreading tumour of any size with its invasive component limited to the bronchial wall, which may extend proximal to the main bronchus, is also classified as T1a.

[c] Solitary adenocarcinoma (not more than 3 cm in greatest dimension), with a predominantly lepidic pattern and not more than 5 mm invasion in greatest dimension in any one focus.

[d] T2 tumours with these features are classified T2a if 4 cm or less, or if size cannot be determined and T2b if greater than 4 cm but not larger than 5 cm.

[e] Most pleural (pericardial) effusions with lung cancer are due to tumour. In a few patients, however, multiple microscopic examinations of pleural (pericardial) fluid are negative for tumour, and the fluid is non-bloody and is not an exudate. Where these elements and clinical judgment dictate that the effusion is not related to the tumour, the effusion should be excluded as a staging descriptor.

[f] This includes involvement of a single non-regional node.

pTNM Pathological Classification

The pT and pN categories correspond to the T and N categories. For pM see page 44.

pN0   Histological examination of hilar and mediastinal lymphadenectomy specimen(s) will ordinarily include 6 or more lymph nodes/stations. Three of these nodes stations should be mediastinal, including the subcarinal nodes and three from N1 nodes/stations. Labelling according to the IASLC chart and table of definitions given in the TNM Supplement is desirable. If all the lymph nodes examined are negative, but the number ordinarily examined is not met, classify as pN0.

Stage

Occult carcinoma	TX	N0	M0
Stage 0	Tis	N0	M0
Stage IA	T1	N0	M0
Stage IA1	T1mi	N0	M0
	T1a	N0	M0
Stage IA2	T1b	N0	M0
Stage IA3	T1c	N0	M0
Stage IB	T2a	N0	M0
Stage IIA	T2b	N0	M0
Stage IIB	T1a-c, T2a, b	N1	M0
	T3	N0	M0
Stage IIIA	T1a-c, T2a, b	N2	M0
	T3	N1	M0
	T4	N0, N1	M0
Stage IIIB	T1a-c, T2a, b	N3	M0
	T3, T4	N2	M0
Stage IIIC	T3, T4	N3	M0
Stage IV	Any T	Any N	M1
Stage IVA	Any T	Any N	M1a, M1b
Stage IVB	Any T	Any N	M1c

Prognostic Factors Grid–Non-Small Cell Lung Carcinoma

Prognostic factors in surgically resected NSCLC

Prognostic Factors	Tumour Related	Host Related	Environment Related
Essential	T category N category Extracapsular nodal extension	Weight loss Performance status	Resection margins Adequacy of mediastinal dissection
Additional	Histological type Grade Vessel invasion Tumour size	Gender Symptom burden	
New and promising	Molecular/biological markers	Quality of life Marital status	

Prognostic risk factors in advanced (locally-advanced or metastatic) NSCLC

Prognostic Factors	Tumour Related	Host Related	Environment Related
Essential	Stage Superior vena cava obstruction (SVCO) Oligometastatic disease Number of sites	Weight loss Performance status	Chemotherapy Targeted therapy
Additional	Number of metastatic sites Pleural effusion Liver metastasis Haemoglobin Lactate dehydrogenase (LDH) Albumin	Gender	
New and promising	Molecular/biological markers	Quality of life Marital status Anxiety/depression	

Source for both tables: *UICC Manual of Clinical Oncology*, Ninth Edition. Edited by Brian O'Sullivan, James D. Brierley, Anil K. D'Cruz, Martin F. Fey, Raphael Pollock, Jan B. Vermorken and Shao Hui Huang. © 2015 UICC. Published 2015 by John Wiley & Sons, Ltd.

Prognostic Factors Grid–Small Cell Lung Carcinoma

Prognostic risk factors in SCLC

Prognostic Factors	Tumour Related	Host Related	Environment Related
Essential	Stage	Performance status Age Comorbidity	Chemotherapy Thoracic radiotherapy Prophylactic cranial radiotherapy
Additional	LDH Alkaline phosphatase Cushing syndrome M0 – mediastinal involvement M1 – number of sites Brain or bone involvement White blood cell count (WBC)/platelet count		
New and promising	Molecular/biological markers		

Source: *UICC Manual of Clinical Oncology*, Ninth Edition. Edited by Brian O'Sullivan, James D. Brierley, Anil K. D'Cruz, Martin F. Fey, Raphael Pollock, Jan B. Vermorken and Shao Hui Huang. © 2015 UICC. Published 2015 by John Wiley & Sons, Ltd.

References

1. Rami-Porta R, Bolejack V, Giroux DJ, et al. The IASLC Lung Cancer Staging Project: the new database to inform the 8th edition of the TNM classification of lung cancer. *J Thorac Oncol* 2014; 9: 1618–1624.
2. Rami-Porta R, Bolejack V, Crowley J, et al. The IASLC Lung Cancer Staging Project: proposals for the revisions of the T descriptors in the forthcoming 8th edition of the TNM classification for lung cancer. *J Thorac Oncol* 2015; 10: 990–1003.
3. Asamura H, Chansky K, Crowley J, et al. The IASLC Lung Cancer Staging Project: proposals for the revisions of the N descriptors in the forthcoming

8th edition of the TNM classification for lung cancer. *J Thorac Oncol* 2015; 10: 1675–1684.

4. Eberhardt WEE, Mitchell A, Crowley J, et al. The IASLC Lung Cancer Staging Project: proposals for the revisions of the M descriptors in the forthcoming 8th edition of the TNM classification for lung cancer. *J Thorac Oncol* 2015; 10: 1515–1522.

5. Goldstraw P, Chansky K, Crowley J, et al. The IASLC Lung Cancer Staging Project: proposals for the revision of the TNM stage grouping in the forthcoming (eighth) edition of the TNM classification for lung cancer. *J Thorac Oncol* 2016;11: 39–51.

6. Nicholson AG, Chansky K, Crowley J, et al. The IASLC Lung Cancer Staging Project: proposals for the revision of the clinical and pathological staging of small cell lung cancer in the forthcoming eighth edition of the TNM classification for lung cancer. *J Thorac Oncol* 2016;11: 300–311.

Executive Editor's Note: This chapter has been reprinted from Wittekind Ch, Compton CC, Brierley J, Sobin LH (eds) UICC TNM Supplement A Commentary on Uniform Use, fourth edition, John Wiley & Sons, Ltd., Oxford, 2012. Where needed, the text has been updated according to the 8th edition of the TNM classification of lung cancer.

3

Site-Specific Explanatory Notes for Lung Tumours

Rules for Classification

The classification applies to all types of carcinoma including non-small cell and small cell carcinoma and to broncho-pulmonary carcinoid tumours. It does not apply to sarcomas and other rare tumours.

Changes to the 7th edition are based upon recommendations from the IASLC Lung Cancer Staging Project.[1-12]

Clinical classification (Pre-treatment clinical classification), designated TNM (or cTNM), is essential to select and evaluate therapy. This is based on evidence acquired before treatment. Such evidence arises from physical examination, imaging (e.g., computed tomography and positron emission tomography), endoscopy (bronchoscopy or oesophagoscopy, with/without ultrasound directed biopsies (EBUS, EUS)), biopsy (including mediastinoscopy, mediastinotomy, thoracocentesis and video-assisted thoracoscopy), as well as surgical exploration, and other relevant examinations such as pleural/pericardial aspiration for cytology.

Pathological classification (post-surgical histopathological classification), designated pTNM, provides the most precise data to estimate prognosis and calculate end results. This is based on the evidence acquired before treatment, supplemented or modified by the additional evidence acquired from surgery and from pathological examination. The pathological assessment of the primary tumour (pT) entails a resection of the primary tumour, or biopsy adequate to evaluate the highest pT category. Removal of nodes adequate to validate the absence of regional lymph node metastasis is required for pN0. The pathological assessment of distant metastasis (pM) entails microscopic examination.

Pathologic staging depends on the proven anatomic extent of disease, whether or not the primary lesion has been completely removed. If a biopsied primary tumour technically cannot be removed, or when it is unreasonable to remove it, the criteria for pathologic classification and staging are satisfied without total removal of the primary cancer if: a) biopsy has confirmed a pT category and there is microscopical confirmation of nodal disease at any level (pN1-3), b) there is microscopical confirmation of the highest N category (pN3), or c) there is microscopical confirmation of pM1.

General Rule 3 states that clinical and pathological data may be combined when only partial information is available in either the pathological classification or the clinical classification, e.g. the classification of a case designated as cT1 pN2 cM1 or pT2 cN0 cM1 would be considered a clinical classification whilst in a case designated pT2 pN2 cM1, cT2 pN3 cM0 or cT2 cN0 pM1 case it would be appropriate to designate a pathological classification.

Histopathologic Type

Table 3.1. 2015 WHO Classification of Lung Tumours [a,b,c]

Histologic Type and Subtypes	ICDO Code
Epithelial tumours	
Adenocarcinoma	8140/3
Lepidic adenocarcinoma[e]	8250/3[d]
Acinar adenocarcinoma	8551/3[d]
Papillary adenocarcinoma	8260/3
Micropapillary adenocarcinoma[e]	8265/3
Solid adenocarcinoma	8230/3
Invasive mucinous adenocarcinoma[e]	8253/3[d]
Mixed invasive mucinous and nonmucinous adenocarcinoma	8254/3[d]
Colloid adenocarcinoma	8480/3
Fetal adenocarcinoma	8333/3
Enteric adenocarcinoma[e]	8144/3
Minimally invasive adenocarcinoma[e]	
Nonmucinous	8256/3[d]
Mucinous	8257/3[d]
Preinvasive lesions	
Atypical adenomatous hyperplasia	8250/0[d]
Adenocarcinoma in situ[e]	
Nonmucinous	8250/2[d]
Mucinous	8253/2[d]
Squamous cell carcinoma	8070/3
Keratinizing squamous cell carcinoma[e]	8071/3
Nonkeratinizing squamous cell carcinoma[e]	8072/3
Basaloid squamous cell carcinoma[e]	8083/3
Preinvasive lesion	
Squamous cell carcinoma in situ	8070/2

continued on next page

Table 3.1. *(continued)*

Histologic Type and Subtypes	ICDO Code
Neuroendocrine tumours	
Small cell carcinoma	8041/3
Combined small cell carcinoma	8045/3
Large cell neuroendocrine carcinoma	8013/3
Combined large cell neuroendocrine carcinoma	8013/3
Carcinoid tumours	
Typical carcinoid tumour	8240/3
Atypical carcinoid tumour	8249/3
Preinvasive lesion	
Diffuse idiopathic pulmonary neuroendocrine cell hyperplasia	8040/0[d]
Large cell carcinoma	8012/3
Adenosquamous carcinoma	8560/3
Sarcomatoid carcinomas	
Pleomorphic carcinoma	8022/3
Spindle cell carcinoma	8032/3
Giant cell carcinoma	8031/3
Carcinosarcoma	8980/3
Pulmonary blastoma	8972/3
Other and unclassified carcinomas	
Lymphoepithelioma-like carcinoma	8082/3
NUT carcinoma[e]	8023/3[d]
Salivary gland-type tumours	
Mucoepidermoid carcinoma	8430/3
Adenoid cystic carcinoma	8200/3
Epithelial-myoepithelial carcinoma	8562/3
Pleomorphic adenoma	8940/0

continued on next page

Neuroendocrine tumours (cont.)	
Papillomas	
Squamous cell papilloma	8052/0
Exophytic	8052/0
Inverted	8053/0
Glandular papilloma	8260/0
Mixed squamous and glandular papilloma	8560/0
Adenomas	
Sclerosing pneumocytoma[e]	8832/0
Alveolar adenoma	8251/0
Papillary adenoma	8260/0
Mucinous cystadenoma	8470/0
Mucous gland adenoma	8480/0
Mesenchymal tumours	
Pulmonary hamartoma	8992/0[d]
Chondroma	9220/0
PEComatous tumours[e]	
Lymphangioleiomyomatosis	9174/1
PEComa, benign[e]	8714/0
Clear cell tumour	8005/0
PEComa, malignant[e]	8714/3
Congenital peribronchial myofibroblastic tumour	8827/1
Diffuse pulmonary lymphangiomatosis	
Inflammatory myofibroblastic tumour	8825/1
Epithelioid hemangioendothelioma	9133/3
Pleuropulmonary blastoma	8973/3
Synovial sarcoma	9040/3
Pulmonary artery intimal sarcoma	9137/3
Pulmonary myxoid sarcoma with EWSR1–CREB1 translocation[e]	8842/3[d]

continued on next page

Table 3.1. *(continued)*

Histologic Type and Subtypes	ICDO Code
Myoepithelial tumours[e]	
Myoepithelioma	8982/0
Myoepithelial carcinoma	8982/3
Lymphohistiocytic tumours	
Extranodal marginal zone lymphomas of mucosa-associated lymphoid tissue (MALT lymphoma)	9699/3
Diffuse large cell lymphoma	9680/3
Lymphomatoid granulomatosis	9766/1
Intravascular large B cell lymphoma[e]	9712/3
Pulmonary Langerhans cell histiocytosis	9751/1
Erdheim–Chester disease	9750/1
Tumours of ectopic origin	
Germ cell tumours	
Teratoma, mature	9080/0
Teratoma, immature	9080/1
Intrapulmonary thymoma	8580/3
Melanoma	8270/3
Meningioma, NOS	9530/0
Metastatic tumours	

[a]*The morphology codes are from the ICDO (Fritz A, Percy C, Jack A, et al. International Classification of Diseases for Oncology. 3rd ed. Geneva: World Health Organization (WHO), 2000). Behavior is coded /0 for benign tumors, /1 for unspecified, borderline or uncertain behavior, /2 for carcinoma in situ and grade III intraepithelial neoplasia, and /3 for malignant tumors.*

[b]*The classification is modified from the previous WHO classification[3] taking into account changes in our understanding of these lesions.*

[c]*This table is reproduced from the 2015 WHO Classification by Travis WD, Brambilla E, Burke AP, Marx A, Nicholson AG. WHO Classification of Tumours of the Lung, Pleura, Thymus and Heart. Lyon: International Agency for Research on Cancer, 2015.*

[d]*These new codes were approved by the International Agency on Cancer Research/WHO Committee for ICDO.*

[e]New terms changed or entities added since 2004 WHO Classification by Travis WD, Brambilla E, Müller-Hermelink HK, Harris CC. Pathology and Genetics: Tumours of the Lung, Pleura, Thymus and Heart. Lyon: IARC, 2004.'

LCNEC, large cell neuroendocrine carcinoma, WHO, World Health Organization; ICDO International Classification of Diseases for Oncology.

From: Travis WD, Brambilla E, Nicholson AG et al. The 2015 World Health Organization Classification of Lung Tumors. Impact of genetic, clinical and radiologic advances since the 2004 classification. J Thorac Oncol 2015; 10: 1243-1260. Used with permission.[13]

Summary Lung

TX   Primary tumour cannot be assessed, or tumour proven by the presence of malignant cells in sputum or bronchial washings but not visualized by imaging or bronchoscopy

T0   No evidence of primary tumour

Tis   Carcinoma *in situ*: Tis (AIS) for adenocarcinoma *in situ*; Tis (SCIS) for squamous cell carcinoma *in situ*.

T1   Tumour 3 cm or less in greatest dimension, surrounded by lung or visceral pleura, without bronchoscopic evidence of invasion more proximal than the lobar bronchus (i.e., not in the main bronchus). The uncommon superficial spreading tumour of any size with its invasive component limited to the bronchial wall, which may extend proximal to the main bronchus, is also classified as T1a.

T1mi Minimally invasive adenocarcinoma

T1a   Tumour 1 cm or less in greatest dimension

T1b   Tumour more than 1 cm but not more than 2 cm in greatest dimension

T1c   Tumour more than 2 cm but not more than 3 cm in greatest dimension

T2   Tumour more than 3 cm but not more than 5 cm; or tumour with any of the following features. T2 tumours with these features are classified T2a if 4 cm or less, or if size cannot be determined; and T2b if greater than 4 cm but not larger than 5 cm.

- Involves main bronchus regardless of distance to the carina, but without involving the carina
- Invades visceral pleura
- Associated with atelectasis or obstructive pneumonitis that extends to the hilar region, either involving part of the lung or the entire lung

T2a   Tumour more than 3 cm but not more than 4 cm in greatest dimension

T2b   Tumour more than 4 cm but not more than 5 cm in greatest dimension

T3   Tumour more than 5 cm but not more than 7 cm in greatest dimension or one that directly invades any of the following: parietal pleura (PL3), chest wall (including superior sulcus tumours), phrenic nerve, parietal pericardium; or associated separate tumour nodule(s) in the same lobe as the primary

T4   Tumour more than 7 cm or one that invades any of the following: diaphragm, mediastinum, heart, great vessels, trachea, recurrent laryngeal nerve, oesophagus, vertebral body, carina; separate tumour nodule(s) in a different ipsilateral lobe to that of the primary

N – Regional Lymph Nodes

NX   Regional lymph nodes cannot be assessed

N0   No regional lymph node metastasis

N1   Metastasis in ipsilateral peribronchial and/or ipsilateral hilar lymph nodes and intrapulmonary nodes, including involvement by direct extension

N2 Metastasis in ipsilateral mediastinal and/or subcarinal lymph node(s)

N3 Metastasis in contralateral mediastinal, contralateral hilar, ipsilateral or contralateral scalene, or supraclavicular lymph node(s)

M – Distant Metastasis

M0 No distant metastasis

M1 Distant metastasis

M1a Separate tumour nodule(s) in a contralateral lobe; tumour with pleural nodules or malignant pleural or pericardial effusion. Most pleural (pericardial) effusions with lung cancer are due to tumour. In a few patients, however, multiple microscopic examinations of pleural (pericardial) fluid are negative for tumour, and the fluid is non-bloody and is not an exudate. Where these elements and clinical judgment dictate that the effusion is not related to the tumour, the effusion should be excluded as a staging descriptor.

M1b Single extrathoracic metastasis in a single organ and involvement of a single distant (non-regional) node

M1c Multiple extrathoracic metastases in one or several organs

T Classification

1. Invasion of visceral pleura (T2) is defined as "invasion beyond the elastic layer including invasion to the visceral pleural surface". The use of elastic stains is recommended when this feature is not clear on routine histology.[14] See Atlas of Lung Cancer Staging, page 115, for the definitions and a graphic description of visceral pleural invasion.

2. Tumour with direct invasion of an adjacent lobe, across the fissure or by direct extension at a point where the fissure is deficient, should be classified as T2a unless other criteria assign a higher T category.

3. Invasion of phrenic nerve is classified as T3.

4. Vocal cord paralysis (resulting from involvement of the recurrent branch of the vagus nerve), superior vena caval obstruction, or compression of the trachea or oesophagus may be related to direct extension of the primary tumour or to lymph node involvement. If associated with direct extension of the primary tumour a classification of T4 is recommended. If the primary tumour is peripheral, vocal cord paralysis is usually related to the presence of N2 disease and should be classified as such.

5. T4: the "great vessels" are
    - Aorta
    - Superior vena cava
    - Inferior vena cava
    - Main pulmonary artery (pulmonary trunk)
    - Intrapericardial portions of the right and left pulmonary artery
    - Intrapericardial portions of the superior and inferior right and left pulmonary veins

    Invasion of more distal branches does not qualify for classification as T4

6. The designation of "Pancoast" tumour relates to the symptom complex or syndrome caused by a tumour arising in the superior sulcus of the lung that involves the inferior branches of the brachial plexus (C8 and/or T1) and, in some cases, the stellate ganglion. Some superior sulcus tumours are more anteriorly located, and cause fewer neurological symptoms but encase the subclavian vessels. The extent

of disease varies in these tumours, and they should be classified according to the established rules. If there is evidence of invasion of the vertebral body or spinal canal, encasement of the subclavian vessels, or unequivocal involvement of the superior branches of the brachial plexus (C8 or above), the tumour is then classified as T4. If no criteria for T4 disease are present, the tumour is classified as T3.

7. Direct extension to parietal pericardium is classified T3 and to visceral pericardium, T4.

8. Tumour extending to rib is classified as T3.

9. The uncommon superficial spreading tumour of any size with its invasive component limited to the bronchial wall, which may extend proximal to the main bronchus, is classified as T1a.

10. The classification of additional tumour nodules in lung cancer depends upon their histological appearances. a) In most situations in which additional tumour nodules are found in association with a lung primary these are metastatic nodules, with identical histological appearances to that of the primary tumour. If limited to the lobe of the primary tumour such tumours are classified as T3, when found in other ipsilateral lobes are designated as T4 and if found in the contralateral lung are designated M1a. b) Multiple tumours may be considered to be synchronous primaries if they are of different histological cell types. Multiple tumours of similar histological appearance should only be considered to be synchronous primary tumours if in the opinion of the pathologist, based on features such as differences in morphology, immunohistochemistry and/or molecular studies, or, in the case of squamous cancers, are associated with carcinoma in situ, they represent differing sub-types of the same histopathological cell type.

Such cases should also have no evidence of mediastinal nodal metastases or of nodal metastases within a common nodal drainage. These circumstances are most commonly encountered when dealing with either bronchioloalveolar carcinomas or adenocarcinomas of mixed subtype with a bronchioloalveolar component. Multiple synchronous primary tumours should be staged separately. The highest T category and stage of disease should be assigned and the multiplicity or the number of tumours should be indicated in parenthesis, e.g. T2(m) or T2. This distinction may require histopathological confirmation of cell type from more than one tumour nodule, where clinically appropriate.

Executive Editor's Note: *Please, see Chapter 5 for additional recommendations on how to classify lung cancers with multiple lesions.*

In the above classification lung differs from other sites in the application of General Rule 5 as the classification of additional tumour nodules applies not only to grossly recognizable tumours but also those that are microscopic or otherwise only discovered on pathological examination, a not unusual finding in lung cancer.

11. Invasion into mediastinal fat is T4. However, if such invasion is clearly limited to fat within the hilum, classification as T2a or T2b is appropriate, depending upon size, unless other features dictate a higher T category.

N Classification

1. The regional lymph nodes are the intrathoracic, scalene, and supraclavicular nodes.
2. The International Association for the Study of Lung Cancer

(IASLC) lymph node definitions are now the recommended means of describing regional lymph node involvement for lung cancers[15] (see Table 3.2 and Figure 3.1). In this nomenclature ipsilateral or contralateral node involvement in #1 would be classified as N3. Involvement of mediastinal nodes, if limited to the midline stations or ipsilateral stations (#2-9), would be classified as N2. Involvement of #10-14 if ipsilateral would be classified as N1. Contralateral involvement of # 2, 4, 5, 6, 8, 9, 10-14 would be classified as N3.

3. Direct extension of the primary tumour into lymph nodes is classified as lymph node metastasis.

4. The IASLC nodal chart has been adopted as the new international chart for the documentation of nodal stations at clinical or pathological staging where detailed assessment of nodes has been made, usually by invasive techniques or at thoracotomy. The concept of nodal zones was suggested in the 7th edition of the TNM classification of lung cancer as a simpler, more utilitarian system for clinical staging where surgical exploration of lymph nodes has not been performed. An exploratory analysis suggested that nodal extent could be grouped into three categories with differing prognoses: i) involvement of a single N1 zone, designated as N1a, ii) involvement of more than one N1 zone, designated as N1b, or a single N2 zone, designated N2a, and iii) involvement of more than one N2 zone, designated as N2b. It was suggested that radiologists, clinicians and oncologists use the classification prospectively, where more detailed data on nodal stations is not available, to assess the utility of such a classification for future revision.

Executive Editor's Note: *For the 8th edition, quantification of nodal disease has been based on the number of nodal stations*

Table 3.2. IASLC Nodal Definitions.

Nodal station	Description	Definition
#1 (Left/ Right)	Low cervical, supraclavicular and sternal notch nodes	<u>Upper border</u>: lower margin of cricoid cartilage <u>Lower border</u>: clavicles bilaterally and, in the midline, the upper border of the manubrium **#L1 and #R1 limited by the midline of the trachea.**
#2 (Left/ Right)	Upper paratracheal nodes	2R: <u>Upper border</u>: apex of lung and pleural space and, in the midline, the upper border of the manubrium <u>Lower border</u>: intersection of caudal margin of innominate vein with the trachea 2L: <u>Upper border</u>: apex of the lung and pleural space and, in the midline, the upper border of the manubrium <u>Lower border</u>: superior border of the aortic arch **As for #4, in #2 the oncologic midline is along the left lateral border of the trachea.**
#3	Pre-vascular and retrotracheal nodes	3a: Prevascular **On the right** <u>upper border:</u> apex of chest <u>lower border:</u> level of carina <u>anterior border:</u> posterior aspect of sternum <u>posterior border:</u> anterior border of superior vena cava **On the left** <u>upper border:</u> apex of chest <u>lower border:</u> level of carina <u>anterior border:</u> posterior aspect of sternum <u>posterior border:</u> left carotid artery 3p: Retrotracheal <u>upper border:</u> apex of chest <u>lower border:</u> carina

continued on next page

#4 (Left/ Right)	Lower paratracheal nodes	4R: includes right paratracheal nodes, and pretracheal nodes extending to the left lateral border of trachea <u>upper border</u>: intersection of caudal margin of innominate vein with the trachea <u>lower border</u>: lower border of azygos vein
		4L: includes nodes to the left of the left lateral border of the trachea, medial to the ligamentum arteriosum <u>upper border</u>: upper margin of the aortic arch <u>lower border</u>: upper rim of the left main pulmonary artery
#5	Subaortic (aorto-pulmonary window)	Subaortic lymph nodes lateral to the ligamentum arteriosum <u>upper border</u>: the lower border of the aortic arch <u>lower border</u>: upper rim of the left main pulmonary artery
#6	Para-aortic nodes (ascending aorta or phrenic)	Lymph nodes anterior and lateral to the ascending aorta and aortic arch <u>upper border</u>: a line tangential to the upper border of the aortic arch <u>lower border</u>: the lower border of the aortic arch
#7	Subcarinal nodes	<u>upper border</u>: the carina of the trachea <u>lower border</u>: the upper border of the lower lobe bronchus on the left; the lower border of the bronchus intermedius on the right

continued on next page

Table 3.2. (cont.).

Nodal station	Description	Definition
#8 (Left/ Right)	Para-oesophageal nodes (below carina)	Nodes lying adjacent to the wall of the oesophagus and to the right or left of the midline, excluding subcarinal nodes <u>upper border</u>: the upper border of the lower lobe bronchus on the left; the lower border of the bronchus intermedius on the right <u>lower border</u>: the diaphragm
#9 (Left/ Right)	Pulmonary ligament nodes	Nodes lying within the pulmonary ligament <u>upper border</u>: the inferior pulmonary vein <u>lower border</u>: the diaphragm
#10 (Left/ Right)	Hilar nodes	Includes nodes immediately adjacent to the mainstem bronchus and hilar vessels including the proximal portions of the pulmonary veins and main pulmonary artery <u>upper border:</u> the lower rim of the azygos vein on the right; upper rim of the pulmonary artery on the left <u>lower border</u>: interlobar region bilaterally
#11	Interlobar nodes	Between the origin of the lobar bronchi *#11s: between the upper lobe bronchus and bronchus intermedius on the right *#11i: between the middle and lower lobe bronchi on the right ˙ optional sub-categories
#12	Lobar nodes	Adjacent to the lobar bronchi
#13	Segmental nodes	Adjacent to the segmental bronchi
#14	Sub-segmental nodes	Adjacent to the subsegmental bronchi

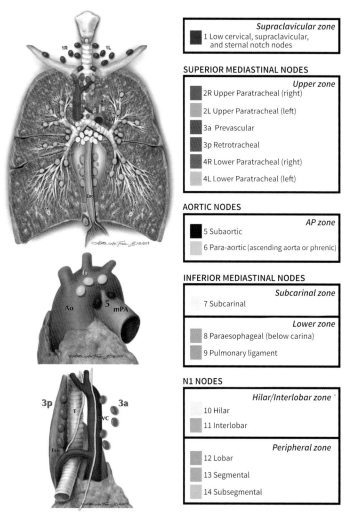

Figure 3.1 International Association for the Study of Lung Cancer Nodal Chart with Stations and Zones. Copyright ©2008 Aletta Ann Frazier, MD.

involved. The survival analyses performed on patients whose tumours were resected and had an adequate intraoperative nodal evaluation revealed four categories with different prognosis: i) involvement of a single N1 station, designated as N1a, ii) involvement of more than one N1 station, designated as N1b, or involvement of one N2 station without N1 disease (skip metastasis), designated as N2a1, iii) involvement of one N2 station with N1 disease, designated as N2a2, and iv) involvement of more than one N2 station, designated N2b. From the analyses of nodal zones and stations, it is evident that the amount of nodal disease has prognostic impact. It is suggested that quantification of nodal disease be made with the available methods at clinical staging, and with systematic nodal dissection at the time of lung resection, either open or video-assisted. Quantifying nodal disease assists physicians in refining prognosis, and in planning therapy and follow-up.

M Classification

1. Pleural/pericardial effusions are classified as M1a, Most pleural (pericardial) effusions with lung cancer are due to tumour. In a few patients, however, multiple microscopical examinations of pleural (pericardial) fluid are negative for tumour, and the fluid is non-bloody and is not an exudate. Where these elements and clinical judgment dictate that the effusion is not related to the tumour, the effusion should be excluded as a descriptor.

2. Tumour foci in the ipsilateral parietal and visceral pleura that are discontinuous from direct pleural invasion by the primary tumour are classified M1a.

3. Pericardial effusion/pericardial nodules are classified as M1a, the same as pleural effusion/nodules.

4. Separate tumour nodules of similar histological appear-

ance are classed as M1a if in the contralateral lung (vide supra regarding synchronous primaries).

5. Distant metastases are classified as M1b if single and M1c if multiple in one or in several organs.

6. Discontinuous tumours outside the parietal pleura in the chest wall or in the diaphragm are classified M1b or M1c depending on the number of lesions.

7. In cases classified as M1b and M1c due to distant metastases it is important to document all of the sites of metastatic disease, whether the sites are solitary or multiple and in addition if the metastases at each site are solitary or multiple.

V Classification

In the lung, arterioles are frequently invaded by cancers. For this reason the V classification is applicable to indicate vascular invasion, whether venous or arteriolar.

Small Cell Carcinoma

The TNM classification and stage grouping should be applied to small cell lung cancer (SCLC). TNM is of significance for prognosis of small cell carcinoma,[6] and has the advantage of providing a uniform detailed classification of tumour spread. TNM should be used when undertaking trials in SCLC. The former categories "limited" and "extensive" for small cell carcinoma have been inconsistently defined and used.

Broncho-Pulmonary Carcinoid Tumours

The TNM classification and stage groupings should be applied to carcinoid tumours, typical and atypical variants.[16]

Isolated Tumour Cells (ITC)

Isolated tumour cells (ITC) are single tumour cells or small clusters of cells not more than 0.2 mm in greatest dimension that are detected by routine histological stains, immunohistochemistry or molecular methods. Cases with ITC in lymph nodes or at distant sites should be classified as N0 or M0, respectively. The same applies to cases with findings suggestive of tumour cells or their components by nonmorphologic techniques such as flow cytometry or DNA analysis.

The following classification of ITC may be used:

N0	No regional lymph node metastasis histologically, no special examination for ITC
N0(i-)	No regional lymph node metastasis histologically, negative morphological findings for ITC
N0(i+)	No regional lymph node metastasis histologically, positive morphological findings for ITC
N0(mol-)	No regional lymph node metastasis histologically, negative nonmorphological findings for ITC
N0(mol+)	No regional lymph node metastasis histologically, positive nonmorphological findings for ITC

Expansion of the R Classification
RX Presence of residual tumour cannot be assessed
R0 Complete resection
All of the following are satisfied:
a) Resection margins confirmed to be clear on microscopy
b) Six nodes/nodal stations removed/sampled for histological examination. These should include three nodes/stations from the mediastinum, one of which should be subcarinal node #7 and three nodes/stations from the hilum or other N1 locations*

R1(cy+)
The requirements for R0 have been met, but pleural lavage cytology (PLC) is positive for malignant cells.

A recent meta-analysis[17] has confirmed that PLC, under-taken immediately on thoracotomy and shown to be positive for cancer cells, has an adverse and independent prognostic impact following complete resection. Such patients may be candidates for adjuvant chemotherapy. Surgeons and pathol-ogists are encouraged to undertake this simple addition to intra-operative staging and collect data on PLC+ve and PLC-ve cases. Where the resection fulfills all of the requirements for classification as a complete resection, R0, but PLC has been performed and is positive, the resection should be classified as R1(cy+).

R1(is)
The requirements for R0 have been met, but *in situ* carcinoma is found at the bronchial resection margin.

R1 Microscopic incomplete resection
Microscopic evidence of residual disease at any of the follow-ing sites:
a) Resection margins
b) Extracapsular extension at margins of resected nodes
c) Positive cytology of pleural/pericardial effusions (R1(cy+))

R2 Macroscopic incomplete resection
Macroscopic evidence of residual disease at any of the fol-lowing sites:
a) Resection margins
b) Extracapsular extension at margins of resected nodes
c) Positive nodes not resected at surgery
d) Pleural/pericardial nodules
*If all resected/sampled lymph nodes are negative, but the number ordinarily included in a lymphadenectomy specimen

is not met, classify as pN0. If resection has been performed, and otherwise fulfils the requirements for complete resection, it should be classified as R0.

A new category, '**R0(un)**', is proposed to document those other features that fall within the proposed category of '**uncertain resection**', i.e. no macroscopic or microscopic evidence of residual disease but any of the following reservations applies:

i) Nodal assessment has been based on less than the number of nodes/stations recommended for complete resection

ii) The highest mediastinal node removed/sampled is positive

References

1. Rami-Porta R, Bolejack V, Giroux DJ et al. The IASLC lung cancer staging project: the new database to inform the eighth edition of the TNM classification of lung cancer. *J Thorac Oncol* 2014; 9: 1618-1624.

2. Rami-Porta R, Bolejack V, Crowley J et al. The IASLC lung cancer staging project: proposals for the revisions of the T descriptors in the forthcoming 8th edition of the TNM classification for lung cancer. *J Thorac Oncol* 2015; 10: 990-1003.

3. Asamura H, Chansky K, Crowley J et al. The IASLC lung cancer staging project: proposals for the revisions of the N descriptors in the forthcoming 8th edition of the TNM classification for lung cancer. *J Thorac Oncol* 2015; 10: 1675-1684.

4. Eberhardt WEE, Mitchell A, Crowley J et al. The IASLC lung cancer staging project: proposals for the revisions of the M descriptors in the forthcoming 8th edition of the TNM classification for lung cancer. *J Thorac Oncol* 2015; 10: 1515-1522.

5. Goldstraw P, Chansky K, Crowley J et al. The IASLC lung cancer staging project: proposals for the revision of the stage grouping in the forthcoming (8th) edition of the TNM classification of lung cancer. *J Thorac Oncol* 2016; 11: 39-51.

6. Nicholson AG, Chansky K, Crowley J et al. The IASLC lung cancer staging project: proposals for the revision of the clinical and pathologic staging of small cell lung cancer in the forthcoming eighth edition of the TNM classification for lung cancer. *J Thorac Oncol* 2016; 11: 300-311.

7. Travis WD, Asamura H, Bankier A et al. The IASLC Lung Cancer Staging Project: proposals for coding T categories for subsolid nodules and

assessment of tumor size in part-solid tumors in the forthcoming eighth edition of the TNM classification of lung cancer. *J Thorac Oncol* 2016; 11: 1204-1223.

8. Detterbeck FC, Franklin WA, Nicholson AG et al. The IASLC Lung Cancer Staging Project: proposed criteria to distinguish separate primary lung cancers from metastatic foci in patients with two lung tumors in the forthcoming eighth edition of the TNM classification for lung cancer. *J Thorac Oncol* 2016; 11: 651-665.

9. Detterbeck FC, Bolejack V, Arenberg DA et al. The IASLC Lung Cancer Staging Project: proposals for the classification of lung cancer with separate tumor nodules in the forthcoming eighth edition of the TNM classification for lung cancer. *J Thorac Oncol* 2016; 11: 681-692.

10. Detterbeck FC, Marom EM, Arenberg DA et al. The IASLC Lung Cancer Staging Project: proposals for the application of TNM staging rules to lung cancer presenting as multiple nodules with ground glass or lepidic features or a pneumonic-type of involvement in the forthcoming eighth edition of the TNM classification. *J Thorac Oncol* 2016; 11: 666-680.

11. Detterbeck FC, Nicholson AG, Franklin WA et al. The IASLC Lung Cancer Staging Project: proposals for revisions of the classification of lung cancers with multiple pulmonary sites of involvement in the forthcoming eighth edition of the TNM classification. *J Thorac Oncol* 2016; 11: 639-650.

12. Detterbeck F, Groome P, Bolejack V et al. The IASLC Lung Cancer Staging Project: methodology and validation used in the development of proposals for revision if the stage classification of non-small cell lung cancer in the forthcoming (eighth) edition of the TNM classification of lung cancer. *J Thorac Oncol* 2016; 11: 1433-1446.

13. Travis WD, Brambilla E, Nicholson AG et al. The 2015 World Health Organization Classification of Lung Tumors. Impact of genetic, clinical and radiologic advances since the 2004 classification. *J Thorac Oncol* 2015; 10: 1243-1260.

14. Travis WD, Brambilla E, Rami-Porta R, et al. Visceral pleural invasion: Pathologic criteria and use of elastic stains: Proposals for the 7th edition of the TNM classification for lung cancer. *J Thorac Oncol* 2008; 3: 1384-1390.

15. Rusch VW, Asamura H, Watanabe H, Giroux DJ, Rami-Porta R, Goldstraw P. The IASLC Lung Cancer Staging Project. A proposal for a new international lymph node map in the forthcoming seventh edition of the TNM classification for lung cancer. *J Thorac Oncol* 2009; 4: 568-577.

16. Travis WD, Giroux DJ, Chansky K, et al. The IASLC Lung Cancer Project: proposals for the inclusion of broncho-pulmonary carcinoid tumors in the

forthcoming (seventh) edition of the TNM classification for lung cancer. *J Thorac Oncol* 2008; 3: 1213-1223.

17. Lim E, Clough R, Goldstraw P et al. Impact of positive pleural lavage cytology on survival of patients having lung resection for non-small-cell lung cancer: An international individual patient data meta-analysis. *J Thorac Cardiovasc Surg* 2010; 139: 1441-1446.

Executive Editor's Note: This chapter has been reprinted from Wittekind Ch, Compton CC, Brierley J, Sobin LH (eds) UICC TNM Supplement A Commentary on Uniform Use, fourth edition, John Wiley & Sons, Ltd., Oxford, 2012. Where needed, the text has been updated according to the 8th edition of the TNM classification of lung cancer.

4

Site-Specific Recommendations for pT and pN Categories

pT – Primary Tumour
The pathological assessment of the primary tumour (pT) entails resection of the primary tumours sufficient to evaluate the highest pT category

pT3 or less
Pathological examination of the primary carcinoma shows *no gross tumour* at the margins of resection (with or without microscopic involvement). pT3 may include additional tumour nodule(s) of similar histological appearance in the lobe of the primary tumour.

pT4
Microscopic confirmation of invasion of any of the following: diaphragm, mediastinum, heart, great vessels, trachea, recurrent laryngeal nerve, oesophagus, vertebral body, carina *or* microscopic confirmation of separate tumour nodule(s) of similar histological appearance in another ipsilateral lobe (not the lobe of the primary tumour)

pN – Regional Lymph Nodes
There are no evidence-based guidelines regarding the number

of lymph nodes to be removed at surgery for adequate staging. However, adequate N staging is generally considered to include sampling or dissection of lymph nodes from stations 2R, 4R, 7, 10R and 11R for right-sided tumours, and stations 5, 6, 7, 10L and 11L for left-sided tumours. Station 9 lymph nodes should also be evaluated for lower lobe tumours. The more peripheral lymph nodes at stations 12-14 are usually evaluated by the pathologist in lobectomy or pneumonectomy specimens but may be separately removed when sublobar resections (e.g. segmentectomy) are performed. These should be labelled in accordance with the IASLC chart and table of definitions[1] (see table and map on pages 78-81).

The UICC recommends that at least six lymph nodes/stations be removed/sampled and confirmed on histology to be free of disease to confer pN0 status. Three of these nodes/stations should be mediastinal, including the subcarinal nodes (#7) and three from N1 nodes/stations.

If all resected/sampled lymph nodes are negative, but the number recommended is not met, classify as pN0. If resection has been performed, and otherwise fulfils the requirements for complete resection, it should be classified as R0.

pN1
Microscopic confirmation of metastasis in ipsilateral peribronchial and/or ipsilateral hilar lymph nodes and intrapulmonary nodes, including involvement by direct extension.

pN2
Microscopic confirmation of metastasis in ipsilateral mediastinal and/or subcarinal lymph node(s).

pN3
Microscopic confirmation of metastasis in contralateral medi-

astinal, contralateral hilar, ipsilateral or contraletaral scalene or supraclavicular lymph node(s).

Reference

1. Rusch VW, Asamura H, Watanabe H, Giroux DJ, Rami-Porta R, Goldstraw P. The IASLC lung cancer staging project. A proposal for a new international lymph node map in the forthcoming seventh edition of the TNM classification for lung cancer. *J Thorac Oncol* 2009; 4: 568-577

5

New Site-Specific Recommendations Proposed by the IASLC

Ramón Rami-Porta, Frank C. Detterbeck, William D. Travis, and Hisao Asamura

The following recommendations for lung cancer classification derive from the analyses of the International Association for the Study of Lung Cancer (IASLC) database, the review of published articles, and a wide international and multidisciplinary consensus. The new categories for adenocarcinoma *in situ* and minimally invasive adenocarcinoma have been accepted by the Union for International Cancer Control (UICC) and by the American Joint Committee on Cancer (AJCC), and will appear in the 8th edition of their respective staging manuals; the other recommendations are included in the 8th edition of the AJCC *Cancer Staging Manual*, but are still under assessment by the UICC. Presumably, they will appear in the 5th edition of the UICC *TNM Supplement – A Commentary on Uniform Use* that is traditionally published after the UICC *TNM Classification of Malignant Tumours*.

New Categories for the New Adenocarcinomas

Adenocarcinoma *in situ* is classified as Tis (AIS) to differentiate it from squamous cell carcinoma *in situ*, which is classified as Tis (SCIS).[1] Tis (AIS) and Tis (SCIS) N0 M0 are stage 0.[2]

Minimally invasive adenocarcinoma is classified as T1mi.[1] T1mi N0 M0 is stage IA1, together with T1a N0 M0.[2]

Measurement of Tumour Size in Part-Solid Non-Mucinous Adenocarcinomas

Part-solid adenocarcinomas present with a solid component and a ground glass opacity on computed tomography (CT). At pathological examination, the solid component usually corresponds to the invasive part; and the ground glass opacity, to the lepidic part. To define the T category by tumour size, only the size of the solid component on CT or the size of the invasive component at pathologic examination are considered, because it is the size of the solid/invasive component that determines prognosis. However, documentation of both the size of the solid component/invasive part and of the whole tumour including the ground glass and lepidic components in radiology and pathology reports, respectively, is recommended.[1]

Measurement of Tumour Size after Induction Therapy

This issue has been rarely discussed in depth before. The recommendation of the IASLC is that tumour size can be measured by multiplying the percentage of viable tumour cells by the total size of the tumour.[1]

Classification of Lung Cancers with Multiple Sites of Involvement

To avoid ambiguity and to facilitate the homogeneous classification of lung cancer with multiple sites of disease, an *ad hoc* sub-committee of the IASLC Staging and Prognostic Factors Committee developed the following recommendations based on the analyses of the IASLC database where data were available, the review of published reports and a wide multidisciplinary and international consensus. The following recommendations apply to grossly identified tumours and to those identified at microscopic examination, and differ depending on the pattern of disease.[3]

- **Synchronous and metachronous primary lung cancers.** Regardless of tumour location, a separate TNM is defined for each tumour. The clinical and pathological criteria to differentiate second primary from related tumours are defined in Table 5.1.[4]

- **Separate tumour nodules with similar histopathologic features (intrapulmonary metastases).** Classification depends on the location of the separate tumour nodule(s): T3 if the separate tumour nodule(s) is(are) in the same lobe of the primary tumour; T4, if located in a different ipsilateral lobe; M1a, if located in the contralateral lung. If there are additional extrathoracic metastases, the tumour will be classified as M1b or M1c depending on the number of metastatic sites. The clinical and pathological criteria to categorise separate tumour nodules (intrathoracic metastasis) are defined in Table 5.2.[5]

- **Multifocal pulmonary adenocarcinoma with ground glass/lepidic features.** Regardless of the location of the tumours, the rule of the highest T with the number (#) or (m) for multiple in parentheses, and an N and an M for all of the multiple tumours collectively applies for these tumours. Table 5.3 shows the clinical and pathologic criteria to define these tumours.[6]

- **Diffuse pneumonic-type lung adenocarcinoma.** A) Single focus of disease. The general TNM classification is applied, with the T category defined by tumour size. B) Multiple foci of disease. Tumour classification is based on the location of the involved areas (including miliary involvement): T3, if located in one lobe; T4, if located in other ipsilateral lobes; M1a, if the contralateral lung is involved, with the

Table 5.1. Criteria for separate versus related pulmonary tumours.[4]

Clinical Criteria*
Tumours may be considered separate primary tumours if: They are clearly of a different histologic type (e.g. squamous carcinoma and adenocarcinoma) by biopsy
Tumours may be considered to be arising from a single tumour source if: Exactly matching breakpoints are identified by comparative genomic hybridization
Relative arguments that favor separate tumours: Different radiographic appearance or metabolic uptake Different biomarker pattern (driver gene mutations) Different rates of growth (if previous imaging is available) Absence of nodal or systemic metastases
Relative arguments that favor a single tumour source: Same radiographic appearance Similar growth patterns (if previous imaging is available) Significant nodal or systemic metastases Same biomarker pattern (and same histotype)
Pathologic Criteria (i.e. after resection)**
Tumours may be considered separate primary tumours if: They are clearly of a different histologic type (e.g. squamous carcinoma and adenocarcinoma) They are clearly different by a comprehensive histologic assessment They are squamous carcinomas that have arisen from carcinoma in situ
Tumours may be considered to be arising from a single tumour source if: Exactly matching breakpoints are identified by comparative | genomic hybridization
Relative arguments that favor separate tumours (to be considered together with clinical factors): Different pattern of biomarkers Absence of nodal or systemic metastases
Relative arguments that favor a single tumour source (to be considered together with clinical factors): Matching appearance on comprehensive histologic assessment Same biomarker pattern Significant nodal or systemic metastases

Note that a comprehensive histologic assessment is not included in clinical staging, as it requires that the entire specimen has been resected.

**Pathologic information should be supplemented with any clinical information that is available.

Table 5.2. Criteria to categorize a lesion as a separate tumour nodule (intrapulmonary metastasis)[3,5]

Clinical Criteria

Tumours should be considered to have a separate tumour nodule(s) if:

There is a solid lung cancer and a separate tumour nodule(s) with a similar solid appearance and with (presumed) matching histologic appearance

- This applies whether or not a biopsy has been performed on the lesions, provided that there is strong suspicion that the lesions are histologically identical

- This applies whether or not there are sites of extrathoracic metastases

AND provided that:

The lesions are NOT judged to be synchronous primary lung cancers

The lesions are NOT multifocal GG/L lung cancer (multiple nodules with ground glass/lepidic features) or pneumonic-type of lung cancer

Pathologic Criteria

Tumours should be considered to have a separate tumour nodule(s) (intrapulmonary metastasis) if:

There is a separate tumour nodule(s) of cancer in the lung with a similar histologic appearance to a primary lung cancer

AND provided that:

The lesions are NOT judged to be synchronous primary lung cancers
The lesions are NOT multiple foci of LPA, MIA, AIS

Note: a radiographically solid appearance and the specific histologic subtype of solid adenocarcinoma denote different things.

AIS, adenocarcinoma in situ; GG/L, ground glass/lepidic; LPA, lepidic predominant adenocarcinoma; MIA, minimally invasive adenocarcinoma

Table 5.3. Criteria identifying multifocal ground glass/lepidic lung adenocarcinoma.[6]

Clinical Criteria

Tumours should be considered multifocal GG/L lung adenocarcinoma if:

There are multiple sub-solid nodules (either pure ground glass or part-solid), with at least one suspected (or proven) to be cancer

- This applies whether or not a biopsy has been performed of the nodules
- This applies if the other nodules(s) are found on biopsy to be AIS, MIA, or LPA
- This applies if a nodule has become >50% solid but is judged to have arisen from a GGN, provided there are other sub-solid nodules
- GGN lesions <5mm or lesions suspected to be AAH are not counted

Pathologic Criteria

Tumours should be considered multifocal GG/L lung adenocarcinoma if:

There are multiple foci of LPA, MIA, or AIS

- This applies whether a detailed histologic assessment (i.e. proportion of subtypes, etc.) shows a matching or different appearance
- This applies if one lesion(s) is LPA, MIA or AIS and there are other sub-solid nodules of which a biopsy has not been performed.
- This applies whether the nodule(s) are identified preoperatively or only on pathologic examination
- Foci of AAH are not counted

Note: a radiographically solid appearance and the specific histologic subtype of solid adenocarcinoma denote different things.
AIS, adenocarcinoma in situ; GG/L, ground glass/lepidic; LPA, lepidic predominant adenocarcinoma; MIA, minimally invasive adenocarcinoma

T category defined by the largest tumour. C) If tumour size is difficult to determine: T4 applies if there is evidence of involvement of another ipsilateral lobe. In all circumstances, the N category should apply to all pulmonary sites and the appropriate M category should be applied depending on the number and location of metastases. The clinical and pathological criteria to define these tumours are shown in Table 5.4.[6]

The basic radiographic and pathologic features, the recommended TNM classification and the conceptual view of the four patterns of lung cancer with multiple sites of involvement are summarised in Table 5.5.

Quantification of Nodal Disease

Quantification of nodal disease has prognostic impact. For the 7th edition of the TNM classification of lung cancer, quantification of nodal disease was based on the number of involved nodal zones.[7] For the 8th edition, it is based on the number of involved nodal stations.[8] Both criteria separate groups of tumours with statistically significant differences. However, both were based on pathological findings of the lymphadenectomy specimen that could not be validated at clinical staging. The recommendation from the IASLC is to quantify nodal disease at pathological staging because it allows the refinement of postoperative prognosis and assists in making decisions on adjuvant therapy, but also to try to quantify it at clinical staging with the available means. The subclassification of nodal disease based on the number of involved nodal stations is as follows:

- N1a: single station N1
- N1b: multiple station N1
- N2a1: single station N2 without N1 disease (skip metastasis)

Table 5.4. Criteria identifying the pneumonic-type of adenocarcinoma.[6]

Clinical Criteria

Tumours should be considered pneumonic-type of adenocarcinoma if:

The cancer manifests in a regional distribution, similar to a pneumonic infiltrate or consolidation

- This applies whether there is one confluent area or multiple regions of disease. The region(s) may be confined to one lobe, in multiple lobes, or bilateral, but should involve a regional pattern of distribution.

- The involved areas may appear to be ground glass, solid consolidation or a combination thereof.

- This can be applied when there is compelling suspicion of malignancy whether or not a biopsy has been performed of the area(s).

- This should not be applied to discrete nodules (i.e. GG/L nodules)

- This should not be applied to tumours causing bronchial obstruction with resultant obstructive pneumonia or atelectasis

Pathologic Criteria

Tumours should be considered pneumonic-type of adenocarcinoma if:

There is diffuse distribution of adenocarcinoma throughout a region(s) of the lung, as opposed to a single well-demarcated mass or multiple discrete well-demarcated nodules

- This typically involves an invasive mucinous adenocarcinoma, although a mixed mucinous and non-mucinous pattern may occur.

- The tumour may show a heterogeneous mixture of acinar, papillary and micropapillary growth patterns, although it is usually lepidic predominant.

Note: a radiographically solid appearance and the specific histologic subtype of solid adenocarcinoma denote different things.

GG/L, ground glass/lepidic

Table 5.5. Schematic summary of patterns of disease and TNM classification of patients with lung cancer with multiple pulmonary sites of involvement.[3]

	Second Primary Lung Cancer	Separate Tumour Nodule (Intrapulmonary metastasis)	Multifocal GG/L Nodules	Pneumonic-Type of Adenocarci-noma
Imaging features	Two or more distinct masses with imaging characteristics of lung cancer (e.g. spiculated)	Typical lung cancer (e.g. solid, spiculated) with separate solid nodule	Multiple ground glass or part-solid nodules	Patchy areas of ground glass and consolidation
Pathologic features	Different histotype or different morphology by comprehensive histologic assessment	Distinct masses with the same morphologic features by comprehensive histologic assessment	Adenocarcinomas with prominent lepidic component (typically varying degrees of AIS, MIA, LPA)	Same histologic features throughout (most often invasive mucinous adenocarcinoma)
TNM classification	Separate cTNM and pTNM for each cancer	Location of separate nodule relative to primary site determines if T3, T4 or M1a; single N and M	T based on highest T lesion with (#/m) indicating multiplicity; single N and M	T based on size or T3 if in single lobe, T4 or M1a if in different ipsilateral or contralateral lobes; single N and M
Conceptual view	Unrelated tumours	Single tumour, with intrapulmonary metastasis	Separate tumours, albeit with similarities	Single tumour, diffuse pulmonary involvement

AIS, adenocarcinoma in situ; GG/L, ground glass/lepidic; LPA, lepidic-predominant adenocarcinoma; MIA, minimally invasive adenocarcinoma; p, pathologic; TNM, tumour, node, metastasis.

- N2a2: single station N2 with N1 disease
- N2b: multiple station N2

Prognosis worsens as the number of involved nodal stations increases, but N1b and N2a1 have the same prognosis.[8]

References

1. Travis WD, Asamura H, Bankier A et al. The IASLC Lung Cancer Staging Project: proposals for coding T categories for subsolid nodules and assessment of tumor size in part-solid tumors in the forthcoming eighth edition of the TNM classification of lung cancer. *J Thorac Oncol* 2016; 11: 1204-1223.
2. Goldstraw P, Chansky K, Crowley J et al. The IASLC Lung Cancer Staging Project: proposals for the revision of the stage grouping in the forthcoming (8th) edition of the TNM classification of lung cancer. *J Thorac Oncol* 2016; 11: 39-51.
3. Detterbeck FC, Nicholson AG, Franklin WA et al. The IASLC Lung Cancer Staging Project: summary of proposals for revisions of the classification of lung cancers with multiple pulmonary sites of involvement in the forthcoming eighth edition of the TNM classification. *J Thorac Oncol* 2016; 11:539-650.
4. Detterbeck FC, Franklin WA, Nicholson AG et al. The IASLC Lung Cancer Staging Project: background data and proposed criteria to distinguish separate primary lung cancers from metastatic foci in patients with two lung tumors in the forthcoming eighth edition of the TNM classification for lung cancer. *J Thorac Oncol* 2016; 11: 651-665.
5. Detterbeck FC, Bolejack V, Arenberg DA et al. The IASLC Lung Cancer Staging Project: background data and proposals for the classification of lung cancer with separate tumor nodules in the forthcoming eighth edition of the TNM classification for lung cancer. *J Thorac Oncol* 2016; 11: 681-692.
6. Detterbeck FC, Marom EM, Arenberg DA et al. The IASLC Lung Cancer Staging Project: background data and proposals for the application of TNM staging rules to lung cancer presenting as multiple nodules with ground glass or lepidic features or a pneumonic-type of involvement in the forthcoming eighth edition of the TNM classification. *J Thorac Oncol* 2016; 11: 666-680.
7. Rusch VW, Crowley J, Giroux DJ, et al. The IASLC Lung Cancer Staging Project: proposals for the revision of the N descriptors in the forthcoming seventh edition of the TNM classifications for lung cancer. *J Thorac Oncol* 2007; 2: 603-612.
8. Asamura H, Chansky K, Crowley J et al. The IASLC Lung Cancer Staging Project: proposals for the revisions of the N descriptors in the forthcoming 8th edition of the TNM classification for lung cancer. *J Thorac Oncol* 2015; 10: 1675-1684.

6

Atlas of Lung Cancer Staging

T1a, T1b　　　**T1c**

Tumour:
≤1cm

Tumour:
>2cm, ≤3cm

Tumour:
>1cm,
≤2cm

Tumour ≤3cm;
any associated
bronchoscopic
invasion should
not extend
proximal
to the lobar
bronchus

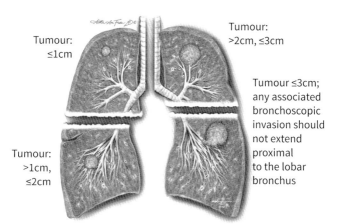

Superficial spreading tumour of
any size with its invasive component
limited to the bronchial wall, which
may extend proximal to the main
bronchus is T1

T2a   T2b

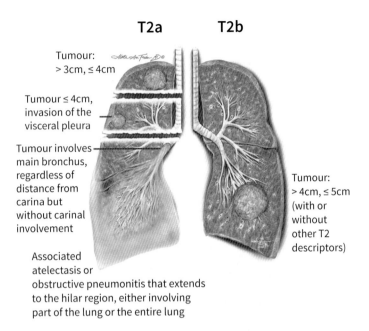

Tumour:
> 3cm, ≤ 4cm

Tumour ≤ 4cm,
invasion of the
visceral pleura

Tumour involves
main bronchus,
regardless of
distance from
carina but
without carinal
involvement

Tumour:
> 4cm, ≤ 5cm
(with or
without
other T2
descriptors)

Associated
atelectasis or
obstructive pneumonitis that extends
to the hilar region, either involving
part of the lung or the entire lung

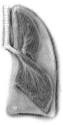

Tumour in the main bronchus
< 2cm from the carina (without
involvement of the carina)
and/or associated atelectasis or
obstructive pneumonitis of
the entire lung

Note: if the tumour is associated with atelectasis or pneumonitis,
it is T2a if lesion ≤ 4cm or if tumour size cannot be measured; it is
T2b if lesion > 4cm, ≤ 5cm.

Chest wall invasion, including
Pancoast tumours without invasion
of vertebral body or spinal canal,
encasement of the subclavian
vessels, or unequivocal involvement
of the superior branches of the
brachial plexus (C8 or above)

T3

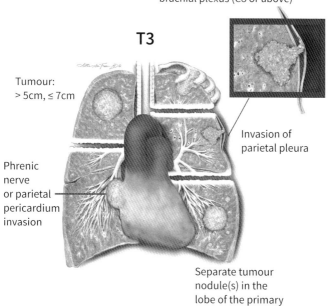

Tumour:
> 5cm, ≤ 7cm

Phrenic
nerve
or parietal
pericardium
invasion

Invasion of
parietal pleura

Separate tumour
nodule(s) in the
lobe of the primary

T4

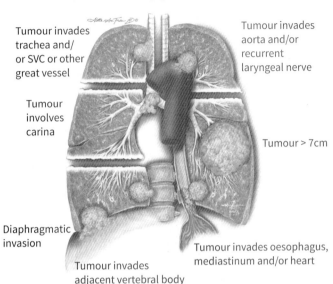

Tumour invades trachea and/or SVC or other great vessel

Tumour involves carina

Tumour invades aorta and/or recurrent laryngeal nerve

Tumour > 7cm

Diaphragmatic invasion

Tumour invades adjacent vertebral body

Tumour invades oesophagus, mediastinum and/or heart

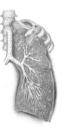

Pancoast tumours with invasion of one or more of the following structures:
- vertebral body or spinal canal
- brachial plexus (C8 or above)
- subclavian vessels

Tumour accompanied by ipsilateral, separate tumour nodules, different lobe

N0   N1

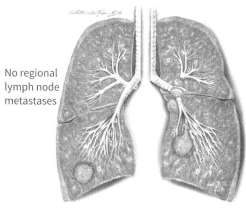

No regional lymph node metastases

Metastasis in ipsilateral intrapulmonary/ peribronchial/ hilar lymph node(s), including nodal involvement by direct extension

N2

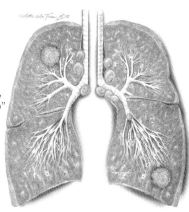

Metastasis in ipsilateral mediastinal and/or subcarinal lymph node(s), including "skip" metastasis without N1 involvement

Metastasis in ipsilateral mediastinal and/or subcarinal lymph node(s) associated with N1 disease

N3

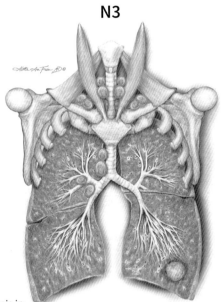

Metastasis in contralateral hilar/ mediastinal/scalene/ supraclavicular lymph node(s)

Metastasis in ipsilateral scalene/supraclavicular lymph node(s)

M1a

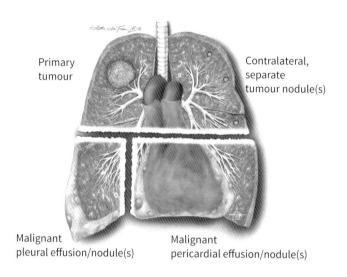

Primary tumour

Contralateral, separate tumour nodule(s)

Malignant pleural effusion/nodule(s)

Malignant pericardial effusion/nodule(s)

Note: when the pleural (pericardial) effusions are negative after multiple microscopic examinations, and the fluid is non-bloody and not an exudate, they should be excluded as a staging descriptor.

M1b

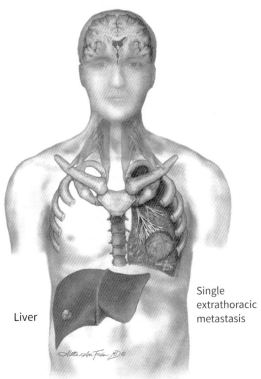

Liver

Single
extrathoracic
metastasis

M1b

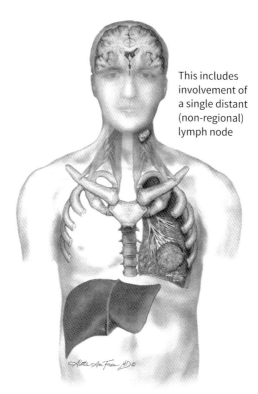

This includes involvement of a single distant (non-regional) lymph node

M1c

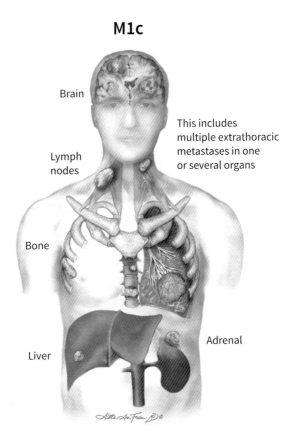

Brain

Lymph nodes

Bone

Liver

This includes multiple extrathoracic metastases in one or several organs

Adrenal

Visceral Pleural Invasion

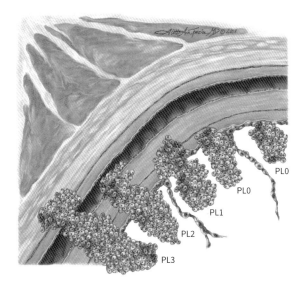

PL0 tumour within the subpleural lung parenchyma or invades superficially into the pleural connective tissue beneath the elastic layer*

PL1 tumour invades beyond the elastic layer

PL2 tumour invades to the pleural surface

PL3 tumour invades into any component of the parietal pleura.

* Note: In the TNM 7th and 8th editions, PL0 is not regarded as a T descriptor and the T category should be assigned on other features. PL1 or PL2 indicate "visceral pleural invasion" i.e. T2a. PL3 indicates invasion of the parietal pleura, i.e. T3.

PART III

PLEURAL MESOTHELIOMA

Acknowledgment: *Used with the permission of the Union for International Cancer Control (UICC), Geneva, Switzerland. The original source for this material is in Brierley JB, Gospodarowicz MK, Wittekind Ch, eds. UICC TNM Classification of Malignant Tumours, 8th edition (2017), published by John Wiley & Sons, Ltd, www.wiley.com.*

7

8th Edition of TNM for Pleural Mesothelioma

Introductory Notes

The classification applies to malignant mesothelioma of pleura.

Each site is described under the following headings:

- Rules for classification with the procedures for assessing T, N, and M categories; additional methods may be used when they enhance the accuracy of appraisal before treatment
- Anatomical subsites where appropriate
- Definition of the regional lymph nodes
- TNM clinical classification
- pTNM pathological classification
- Stage
- Prognostic factors grid

Regional Lymph Nodes

The regional lymph nodes extend from the supraclavicular region to the diaphragm. Direct extension of the primary tumour into lymph nodes is classified as lymph node metastasis.

Pleural Mesothelioma
(ICD-O C38.4)

Rules for Classification

The classification applies only to malignant mesothelioma of the pleura.

There should be histological confirmation of the disease.

Changes in this edition from the seventh edition are based upon recommendations from the International Association for the Study of Lung Cancer (IASLC) Staging Project.[1-5]

The following are the procedures for assessing T, N, and M categories:

T categories	Physical examination, imaging, endoscopy, and/or surgical exploration
N categories	Physical examination, imaging, endoscopy, and/or surgical exploration
M categories	Physical examination, imaging, and/or surgical exploration

Regional Lymph Nodes

The regional lymph nodes are the intrathoracic, internal mammary, scalene, and supraclavicular nodes.

TNM Clinical Classification

T – Primary Tumour

TX Primary tumour cannot be assessed.

T0 No evidence of primary tumour

T1 Tumour involves ipsilateral parietal or visceral pleura only, with or without involvement of visceral, mediastinal or diaphragmatic pleura.

T2 Tumour involves the ipsilateral pleura (parietal or visceral pleura), with at least one of the following:
  • invasion of diaphragmatic muscle
  • invasion of lung parenchyma

T3 Tumour involves ipsilateral pleura (parietal or visceral

pleura), with at least one of the following:
- invasion of endothoracic fascia
- invasion into mediastinal fat
- solitary focus of tumour invading soft tissues of the chest wall
- non-transmural involvement of the pericardium

T4   Tumour involves ipsilateral pleura (parietal or visceral pleura), with at least one of the following:
- chest wall, with or without associated rib destruction (diffuse or multifocal)
- peritoneum (via direct transdiaphragmatic extension)
- contralateral pleura
- mediastinal organs (oesophagus, trachea, heart, great vessels)
- vertebra, neuroforamen, spinal cord
- internal surface of the pericardium (transmural invasion with or without a pericardial effusion)

N – Regional Lymph Nodes

NX   Regional lymph nodes cannot be assessed
N0   No regional lymph node metastasis
N1   Metastases to ipsilateral intrathoracic lymph nodes (includes ipsilateral bronchopulmonary, hilar, subcarinal, paratracheal, aortopulmonary, paraesophageal, peridiaphragmatic, pericardial fat pad, intercostal and internal mammary nodes)
N2   Metastases to contralateral intrathoracic lymph nodes. Metastases to ipsilateral or contralateral supraclavicular lymph nodes

M – Distant Metastasis

M0   No distant metastasis
M1   Distant metastasis

pTNM Pathological Classification
The pT and pN categories correspond to the T and N categories. For pM see page 44.

Stage – Pleural Mesothelioma

Stage IA	T1	N0	M0
Stage IB	T2, T3	N0	M0
Stage II	T1, T2	N1	M0
Stage IIIA	T3	N1	M0
Stage IIIB	T1. T2, T3	N2	M0
	T4	Any N	M0
Stage IV	Any T	Any N	M1

References

1. Rusch VW, Giroux D, Kennedy C et al. Initial analysis of the International Association for the Study of Lung Cancer Mesothelioma database. *J Thorac Oncol* 2012; 7: 1631-1639.
2. Pass H, Giroux D, Kennedy C et al. The IASLC Mesothelioma database: improving staging of a rare disease through international participation. *J Thorac Oncol* 2016; in press.
3. Nowak AK, Chansky K, Rice DC et al. The IASLC Mesothelioma Staging Project: proposals for revisions of the T descriptors in the forthcoming eighth edition of the TNM classification for mesothelioma. *J Thorac Oncol* 2016; in press.
4. Rice D, Chansky K, Nowak A et al. The IASLC Mesothelioma Staging Project: proposals for revisions of the N descriptors in the forthcoming eighth edition of the TNM classification for malignant pleural mesothelioma. *J Thorac Oncol* 2016; in press.
5. Rusch VW, Chansky K, Kindler HL et al. The IASLC Malignant Pleural Mesothelioma Staging Project: proposals for the M descriptors and for the revision of the TNM stage groupings in the forthcoming (eighth) edition of the TNM classification for mesothelioma. *J Thorac Oncol* , 2016; in press.

8

Atlas of
Pleural Mesothelioma Staging

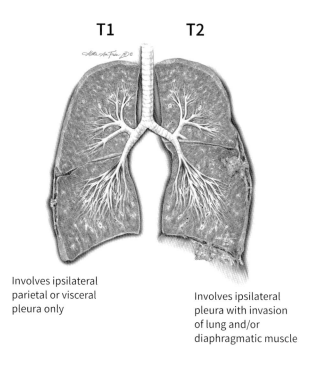

T1

T2

Involves ipsilateral
parietal or visceral
pleura only

Involves ipsilateral
pleura with invasion
of lung and/or
diaphragmatic muscle

T3   T4

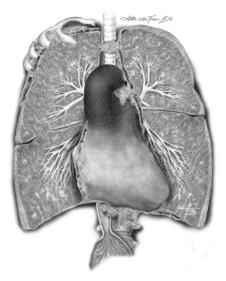

Involves ipsilateral pleura with invasion of the endothoracic fascia, the chest wall (solitary, resectable focus extending into soft tissue),mediastinal fat and/or non-transmural invasion of the pericardium

Involves ipsilateral pleura with diffuse, multifocal invasionof the chest wall, invasion of the contralateral pleura, peritoneum, mediastinal organs, spine, transmural invasion of the pericardium (with or without pericardial effusion) and/or myocardium

N1

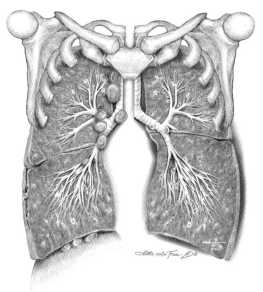

Metastases to ipsilateral intrathoracic lymph nodes (includes ipsilateral bronchopulmonary, hilar, subcarinal, paratracheal, aortopulmonary, para-oesophageal, peridiaphragmatic, pericardial, intercostal and internal mammary lymph nodes)

N2

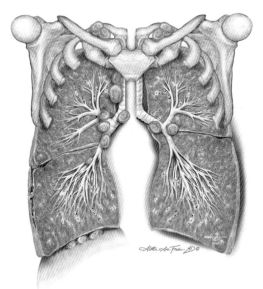

Metastases to contralateral intrathoracic lymph nodes

Metastases to ipsilateral or contralateral supraclavicular lymph nodes

PART IV

THYMIC MALIGNANCIES

Acknowledgment: Used with the permission of the Union for International Cancer Control (UICC), Geneva, Switzerland. The original source for this material is in Brierley JB, Gospodarowicz MK, Wittekind Ch, eds. UICC TNM Classification of Malignant Tumours, 8th edition (2017), published by John Wiley & Sons, Ltd, www.wiley.com.

9

TNM for Thymic Malignancies

Introductory Notes

The classification applies to thymic tumours.
Each site is described under the following headings:

- Rules for classification with the procedures for assessing T, N, and M categories; additional methods may be used when they enhance the accuracy of appraisal before treatment
- Anatomical subsites where appropriate
- Definition of the regional lymph nodes
- TNM clinical classification
- pTNM pathological classification
- Stage
- Prognostic factors grid

Regional Lymph Nodes

The regional lymph nodes extend from the supraclavicular region to the diaphragm. Direct extension of the primary tumour into lymph nodes is classified as lymph node metastasis.

Thymic Tumours
ICD-0-3 C37.9

Rules for Classification

The classification applies to epithelial tumours of the thymus, including thymomas, thymic carcinomas and neuroendocrine tumours of the thymus. It does not apply to sarcomas, lymphomas and other rare tumours.

This classification is new to the 8th edition and is based upon recommendations from the International Association for the Study of Lung Cancer (IASLC) Staging Project and the International Thymic Malignancies Interest Group (ITMIG) (see references).[1–3]

There should be histological confirmation of the disease and division of cases by histological type.

The following are the procedures for assessing T, N, and M categories:

T categories	Physical examination, imaging, endoscopy, and/or surgical exploration
N categories	Physical examination, imaging, endoscopy, and/or surgical exploration
M categories	Physical examination, imaging, and/or surgical exploration

Regional Lymph Nodes

The regional lymph nodes are the anterior (perithymic) lymph nodes, the deep intrathoracic lymph nodes and the cervical lymph nodes.

TNM Clinical Classification

T – Primary Tumour

TX   Primary tumour cannot be assessed.

T0   No evidence of primary tumour

T1   Tumour encapsulated or extending into the mediastinal fat, may involve the mediastinal pleura.

	T1a	No mediastinal pleural involvement
	T1b	Direct invasion of the mediastinal pleura

T2   Tumour with direct involvement of the pericardium (partial or full thickness).

T3   Tumour with direct invasion into any of the following; lung, brachiocephalic vein, superior vena cava, phrenic nerve, chest wall, or extrapericardial pulmonary artery or vein.

T4   Tumour with direct invasion into any of the following; aorta (ascending, arch or descending), arch vessels, intrapericardial pulmonary artery, myocardium, trachea, or oesophagus

N – Regional Lymph Nodes

NX   Regional lymph nodes cannot be assessed

N0   No regional lymph node metastasis

N1   Metastasis in anterior (perithymic) lymph nodes

N2   Metastasis in deep intrathoracic or cervical lymph nodes

M – Distant Metastasis

M0   No pleural, pericardial or distant metastasis

M1   Distant metastasis

    M1a   Separate pleural or pericardial nodule(s)

    M1b   Distant metastasis beyond the pleura or pericardium

TNM Pathological Classification

The pT and pN categories correspond to the T and N categories. For pM see page 44.

Stage –Thymic Tumours

Stage I	T1	N0	M0
Stage II	T2	N0	M0
Stage IIIA	T3	N0	M0
Stage IIIB	T4	N0	M0
Stage IVA	Any T	N1	M0
Stage IVB	Any T	N0, N1	M1a
	Any T	N2	M0, M1a
	Any T	Any N	M1b

References

1. Nicholson AG, Detterbeck FC, Marino M, et al. The IASLC/ITMIG thymic epithelial tumors staging project: proposals for the T component for the forthcoming (8th) edition of the TNM classification of malignant tumors. *J Thorac Oncol* 2014; 9: s73–s80.

2. Kondo K, Van Schil P, Detterbeck FC, et al. The IASLC/ITMIG thymic epithelial tumors staging project: proposals for the N and M components for the forthcoming (8th) edition of the TNM classification of malignant tumors. *J Thorac Oncol* 2014; 9: s81–s87.

3. Detterbeck FC, Stratton K, Giroux D, et al. The IASLC/ITMIG thymic epithelial tumors staging project: proposal for an evidence-based stage classification system for the forthcoming (8th) edition of the TNM classification of malignant tumors. *J Thorac Oncol* 2014; 9: s65–s72.

10

Site-Specific Explanatory Notes for Thymic Malignancies

Frank Detterbeck

Clinical Stage Classification

1. The reliability of imaging characteristics in predicting actual invasion of mediastinal structures has generally not been defined. One must rely on the radiologist's best judgment. An elevated hemidiaphragm should be considered evidence of phrenic nerve involvement.

2. Lymph nodes ≥ 1cm in short axial dimension should be considered involved for purposes of clinical staging; similarly, nodes with PET uptake (if available) should also be considered involved.

3. A surgical exploration without microscopic confirmation of levels of invasion or the nodal status defines the clinical stage. Pathologic stage can be defined if a tumour is completely resected or if invasion of the highest T category is microscopically confirmed along with node sampling.

Pathologic Stage Classification
T Component

1. For pathologic T classification involvement of a particular tissue must be microscopically confirmed. Surgically identified adhesion of the tumour to an adjacent structure does

not affect the T classification if no actual invasion of the adjacent structure is present on microscopic examination.

2. The presence or absence of a capsule or invasion thereof is not a descriptor in the T classification. The International Association for the Study of Lung Cancer-International Thymic Malignancies Interest Group (IASLC-ITMIG) analysis of a large global database demonstrated that these descriptors have no impact on outcomes.[1] This also confirms other studies.[2]

3. The impact of invasion of the mediastinal pleura is unclear. The IASLC-ITMIG database did not demonstrate a difference,[1] but a possible difference is suggested in the Japanese Association for Research on the Thymus (JART) database.[1] A problem with the analysis is that recognition of the mediastinal pleura can be difficult grossly as well as microscopically in the resected specimen. ITMIG recommends routine marking of the mediastinal pleura by the surgeon at the time of resection,[3] and the use of elastin stains is recommended when the mediastinal pleural layer is unclear microscopically.

4. Invasion of the pericardium is classified as T2 whether this is partial or full thickness.[1] The classification is the same whether there is involvement of the parietal and visceral pericardium. (There is no data suggesting a difference in outcomes, and no ability to make this distinction in clinical staging.)

5. While it is recommended that tumour size be recorded, it does not affect the T classification. In the IASLC-ITMIG global database the largest dimension of tumour size had no prognostic impact.

6. The T category is determined by the "level" of invasion. Invasion of structures of a particular T level is counted

regardless whether or not there is invasion of structures of a lower level.

7. While the number of invaded mediastinal structures (of a particular level) appears to affect outcomes, this is not a factor in determining the T category. This is due to some inconsistency and a suspected variable amount of missing information regarding all of the invaded structures in the available data for analysis. It is recommended that not only is the T category recorded, but also all of the specific structures that are invaded.

8. Direct invasion of the pleura or pericardium is distinguished from pleural or pericardial nodules that are separated from the primary tumour mass (see M category notes).

N Component

1. Direct extension of the primary tumour into a lymph node is counted as nodal involvement.[4]

2. During resection of a thymoma with invasion of other structures (i.e. ≥ T2) it is recommended that anterior mediastinal nodes are routinely removed with the specimen, and systematic sampling of deep nodes in encouraged. During resection of a thymic carcinoma systematic resection of both N1 and N2 nodes is recommended. The pathologists should specifically examine and report on the presence of nodal involvement.[3-5] Furthermore, removal and specific notation of any suspicious nodes (either by imaging or intraoperative assessment) is recommended.

3. Nodal involvement is divided into an anterior (perithymic, N1) and deep (N2) category, as detailed in the ITMIG-IASLC node map (Table 10.1, 10.2 and Figures 10.1-10.6).[4,6]

Table 10.1. Anterior Region [N1] (Anterior Mediastinal & Anterior Cervical Nodes).

Region Boundaries	Node Groups[14, 16]	Node Group Boundaries
Sup: hyoid bone Lat (Neck): medial border of carotid sheaths Lat (Chest): mediastinal pleura Ant: sternum Post (Medially): great vessels, pericardium Post (Laterally): phrenic nerve Inf: xiphoid, diaphragm	Low Ant Cervical: pretracheal, paratracheal, peri-thyroid, precricoid/delphian (AAO-HNS / ASHNS level 6 / IASLC level 1)	Sup: inferior border of cricoid Lat: common carotid arteries Inf: superior border of manubrium
	Peri-thymic	Proximity to thymus
	Prevascular (IASLC level 3a)	Sup: apex of chest Ant: posterior sternum Post: anterior SVC Inf: carina
	Paraaortic, ascending aorta, superior phrenic (IASLC level 6)	Sup: line tangential to sup border of aortic arch Inf: inf border of aortic arch
	Supradiaphragmatic/inferior phrenic/pericardial (along inferior poles of thymus)	Sup: inf border of aortic arch Ant: post sternum Post: phrenic nerve (laterally) or pericardium (medially) Inf: diaphragm

Region and node group boundaries adapted directly from definitions established by AAO-HNS, ASHNS and IASLC.

AAO-HNS, American Academy of Otolaryngology - Head and Neck Surgery; ASHNS, American Society for Head and Neck Surgery; IASLC, International Association for the Study of Lung Cancer. Sup, Superior; Ant, Anterior; Inf, inferior; Lat, lateral; Post, posterior; SVC, superior vena cava.

Table 10.2. Deep Region [N2] (Middle Mediastinal and Deep Cervical Nodes.

Region Boundaries	Node Groups[14, 16]	Node Group Boundaries
Sup: level of lower border of cricoid cartilage	Lower jugular (AAO-HNS / ASHNS level 4)	Sup: level of lower border of cricoid cartilage
Anteromedial (neck): lateral border of sternohyoid, medial border of carotid sheath		Anteromedial: lat border of sternohyoid
		Posterolateral: lat border of sternocleidomastoid
		Inf: clavicle
Posterolateral (neck): anterior border of trapezius	Supraclavicular/ venous angle: confluence of internal jugular & subclavian vein (AAO-HNS / ASHNS level 5b)	Sup: level of lower border of cricoid cartilage
		Anteromedial: post border of sternocleidomastoid
Ant (chest): aortic arch, aortopulmonary window–anterior border of SVC		Posterolateral: ant border of trapezius
		Inf: clavicle
	Internal mammary nodes	Proximity to internal mammary arteries
Post (chest): oesophagus	Upper paratracheal (IASLC level 2)	Sup: sup border of manubrium, apices of lungs
Lat (chest): pulmonary hila		Inf: intersection of lower border of innominate vein with trachea; sup border of aortic arch
Inf: diaphragm	Lower paratracheal (IASLC level 4)	Sup: intersection of lower border of innominate vein with trachea; sup border of aortic arch
		Inf: lower border of azygos vein, sup border of left main pulmonary artery

continued on next page

Table 10.2. (cont.)

Region Boundaries	Node Groups[14, 16]	Node Group Boundaries
	Subaortic/aortopulmonary window (IASLC level 5)	Sup: inf border of aortic arch Inf: sup border of left main pulmonary artery
	Subcarinal (IASLC level 7)	Sup: carina Inf: upper border of lower lobe bronchus on the left; lower border of the bronchus intermedius on the right
	Hilar (IASLC level 10)	Sup: lower rim of azygos vein on right, upper rim of pulmonary artery on left Inf: interlobar region bilaterally

Region and node group boundaries adapted directly from definitions established by AAO-HNS, ASHNS and IASLC.

AAO-HNS, American Academy of Otolaryngology - Head and Neck Surgery; ASHNS, American Society for Head and Neck Surgery; IASLC, International Association for the Study of Lung Cancer. Sup, Superior; Ant, Anterior; Inf, inferior; Lat, lateral; Post, posterior; SVC, superior vena cava.

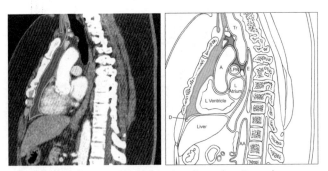

Figure 10.1. Mediastinum, Sagittal Section. Tr=trachea; E=esophagus; LPA=left pulmonary artery; A=aorta; D=diaphragm.

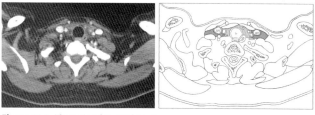

Figure 10.2. Thoracic Inlet, Axial Section.
CCA=common carotid artery; IJV=internal jugular vein; Tr=trachea;
Clav=clavicle; E=esophagus.

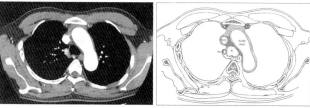

Figure 10.3. Paraaortic Level, Axial Section.
SVC=superior vena cava; E=esophagus; Tr=trachea.

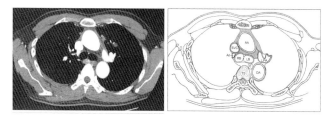

Figure 10.4. AP Window Level, Axial Section.
Note: deep region includes aortopulmonary window nodes.
AA=ascending aorta; DA=descending aorta; LPA=left pulmonary artery;
SVC=superior vena cava; Az=azygos vein; RB=right main bronchus;
LB=left main bronchus.

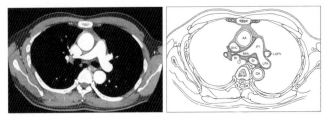

Figure 10.5. Carina Level, Axial Section.
Note: deep region includes aortopulmonary window nodes.
AA=ascending aorta; DA=descending aorta; PT=pulmonary trunk; LPA=left pulmonary artery; RPA=right pulmonary artery; SVC=superior vena cava; LSPV=left superior pulmonary vein; BR=bronchus; E=esophagus.

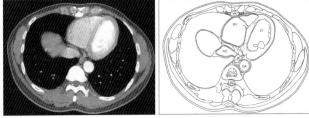

Figure 10.6. Diaphragm Level, Axial Section.
RV=right ventricle; LV=left ventricle; IVC=inferior vena cava; DA=descending aorta; E=esophagus.

M Component

1. Pleural or pericardial nodules that are separate from the primary tumor mass are classified as M1a.[4]
2. Discrete intraparenchymal nodules in the lung are classified as M1b. These are nodules of tumor that are surrounded by normal lung (i.e. not contiguous with the visceral pleura or intraparenchymal tumor that represents direct invasion by the primary tumor mass).[4]

Resection (R) Status

The thymus is generally surrounded by loose areolar tissue, which is prone to disruption either during resection or during handling of the specimen. Furthermore, a thymectomy specimen often includes no tissues that inherently orient the specimen. Therefore, specific attention is necessary to intraoperative marking, specimen handling and orientation, and communication between the surgeon and pathologists in order to accurately report the margin status of resected tumors.[3]

1. It is suggested that immediate intraoperative marking of the specimen be performed to define areas of concern, areas of tissue disruption during handling that do not represent true margins, and specific surfaces (e.g. the right or left mediastinal pleura, areas adjacent to the innominate vein or pericardium)
2. It is recommended that the resected specimen be clearly oriented and that the margin status of specific surfaces be examined and reported (e.g. anterior, posterior, right, left, adjacent to pericardium etc.).[3] ITMIG suggests placing the specimen on a "mediastinal board" that makes the relationship of different parts of the specimen to adjacent structures clear (Figure 10.7).
3. It is recommended that the surgeon and the pathologist communicate at the time of resection about orientation and areas of particular concern
4. The distance to the nearest margin should be reported in mm whenever the margin is ≤ 3mm.

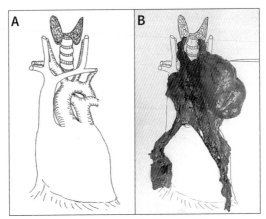

Figure 10.7. A) Mediastinal board and B) example of specimen orientation.

References

1. Nicholson A, Detterbeck C, Marino M, et al. The ITMIG/IASLC Thymic Epithelial Tumors Staging Project: proposals for the T component for the forthcoming (8th) edition of the TNM classification of malignant tumors. *J Thorac Oncol.* 2014; 9 (9, Suppl 2):S73-S80.

2. Marchevsky AM, McKenna Jr RJ, Gupta R. Thymic epithelial neoplasms: a review of current concepts using an evidence-based pathology approach. *Hematol Oncol Clin North Am.* 2008;22(3):543-562.

3. Detterbeck F, Moran C, Huang J, et al. Which way is up? Policies and procedures for surgeons and pathologicsts regarding resection specimens of thymic malignancy. *J Thorac Oncol.* 2011; 6(7 Suppl 3): S1730-S1738.

4. Kondo K, Van Schil P, Detterbeck F, et al. The IASLC/ITMIG Thymic Epithelial Tumors Staging Project: proposals for the N and M components for the forthcoming (8th) edition of the TNM classification of malignant tumors *J Thorac Oncol.* 2014; 9(9, Suppl 2):S81-S87.

5. Park IK, Kim YT, Jeon JH, et al. Importance of lymph node dissection in thymic carcinoma. *Ann Thorac Surg.* 2013; 96(3):1025-1032.

6. Bhora F, Chen D, Detterbeck F, et al. The ITMIG/IASLC Thymic Epithelial Tumors Staging Project: a proposed lymph node map for thymic epithelial tumors in the forthcoming (8th) edition of the TNM classification for malignant tumors. *J Thorac Oncol.* 2014; 9 (9, Suppl 2):S88-S96.

11

Atlas of
Thymic Malignancies Staging

Axial #1

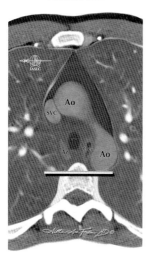

Axial #2

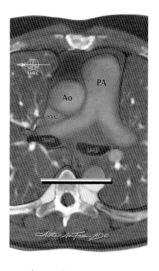

Ao: aorta
PA: pulmonary artery
SVC: superior vena cava
T: trachea
Az: azygos vein
Oes: oesophagus
RMB: right main bronchus
LMB: left main bronchus

Prevascular compartment
Visceral compartment
Paravertebral compartment
Visceral-paravertebral boundary

Axial #3

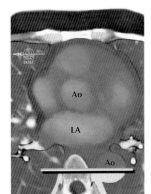

Sagittal

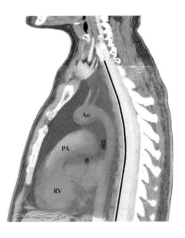

▨ Prevascular compartment	Ao: aorta
▨ Visceral compartment	PA: pulmonary artery
▨ Paravertebral compartment	LA: left atrium
▬ Visceral-paravertebral boundary	RV: right ventricle

Stage I
T1N0M0

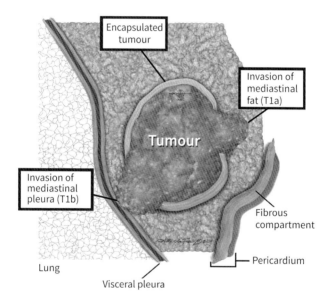

Stage II
T2N0M0

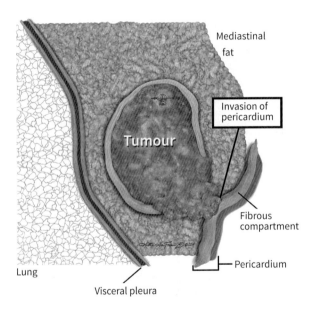

Mediastinal fat

Invasion of pericardium

Tumour

Fibrous compartment

Pericardium

Lung

Visceral pleura

Stage IIIA
T3N0M0

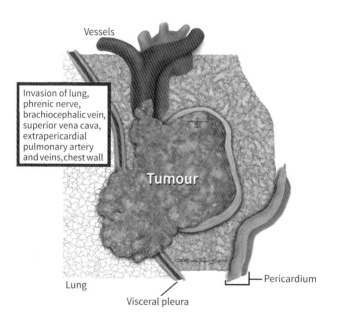

Vessels

Invasion of lung, phrenic nerve, brachiocephalic vein, superior vena cava, extrapericardial pulmonary artery and veins, chest wall

Tumour

Lung

Visceral pleura

Pericardium

Stage IIIB

T4N0M0

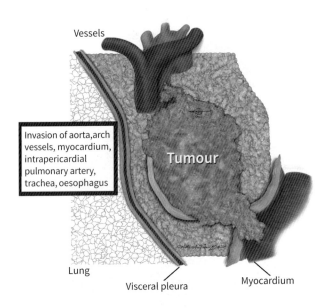

Vessels

Invasion of aorta, arch vessels, myocardium, intrapericardial pulmonary artery, trachea, oesophagus

Tumour

Lung

Visceral pleura

Myocardium

Stage IVA
Any T N1M0;
any T N0-1 M1a

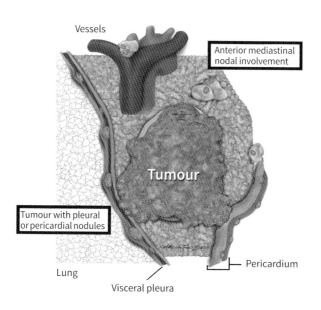

Vessels

Anterior mediastinal nodal involvement

Tumour

Tumour with pleural or pericardial nodules

Pericardium

Lung

Visceral pleura

Stage IVB

Any T N2 M0-1a;
any T, any N, M1b

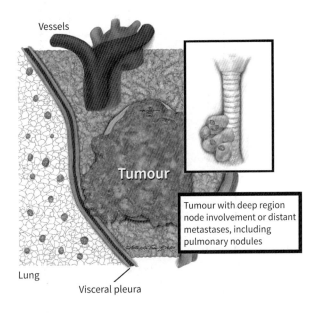

Vessels

Tumour

Tumour with deep region node involvement or distant metastases, including pulmonary nodules

Lung

Visceral pleura

PART V

CARCINOMA OF THE OESOPHAGUS AND OF OESOPHAGOGASTRIC JUNCTION

Acknowledgment: Used with the permission of the Union for International Cancer Control (UICC), Geneva, Switzerland. The original source for this material is in Brierley JB, Gospodarowicz MK, Wittekind Ch, eds. UICC TNM Classification of Malignant Tumours, 8th edition (2017), published by John Wiley & Sons, Ltd, www.wiley.com. There are some differences between the published 8th editions of the TNM classification of carcinoma of the oesophagus and of the oesophagogastric junction published by the UICC and the American Joint Committee on Cancer. The Editorial Addendum following this chapter explains these differences.

12

8th Edition of TNM for Carcinoma of the Oesophagus and of the Oesophagogastric Junction

Rules for Classification

The classification applies only to carcinomas and includes adenocarcinomas of the oesophagogastric/gastroesophageal junction. There should be histological confirmation of the disease and division of cases by topographic localization and histological type. A tumour the epicentre of which is within 2 cm of the **oesophagogastric junction** and also extends into the oesophagus is classified and staged using the oesophageal scheme. Cancers involving the oesophagogastric junction (OGJ) whose epicentre is within the proximal 2 cm of the cardia (Siewert types I/II) are to be staged as oesophageal cancers.

The following are the procedures for assessing T, N, and M categories:

T categories	Physical examination, imaging, endoscopy, (including bronchoscopy), and/or surgical exploration
N categories	Physical examination, imaging, and/or surgical exploration
M categories	Physical examination, imaging, and/or surgical exploration

Anatomical Subsites

1. Cervical oesophagus (C15.0): this commences at the lower border of the cricoid cartilage and ends at the thoracic inlet (suprasternal notch), approximately 18 cm from the upper incisor teeth.
2. Intrathoracic oesophagus
   a) The upper thoracic portion (C15.3) extending from the thoracic inlet to the level of the tracheal bifurcation, approximately 24 cm from the upper incisor teeth.
   b) The mid-thoracic portion (C15.4) is the proximal half of the oesophagus between the tracheal bifurcation and the oesophagogastric junction. The lower level is approximately 32 cm from the upper incisor teeth.
   c) The lower thoracic portion (C15.5), approximately 8 cm in length (includes abdominal oesophagus), is the distal half of the oesophagus between the tracheal bifurcation and the oesophagogastric junction. The lower level is approximately 40 cm from the upper incisor teeth.
3. Oesophagogastric junction (C16.0). Cancers involving the oesophagogastric junction (OGJ) whose epicentre is within the proximal 2 cm of the cardia (Slewert types I/II) are to be staged as oesophageal cancers. Cancers whose epicentre is more than 2 cm distal from the OGJ will be staged using the Stomach Cancer TNM and Stage even if the OGJ is involved.

Regional Lymph Nodes

The regional lymph nodes, irrespective of the site of the primary tumour, are those in the oesophageal drainage area including coeliac axis nodes and paraesophageal nodes in the neck but not the supraclavicular nodes.

TNM Clinical Classification
T – Primary Tumour

TX   Primary tumour cannot be assessed

T0   No evidence of primary tumour

Tis   Carcinoma *in situ*/high-grade dysplasia

T1   Tumour invades lamina propria, muscularis mucosae, or submucosa

    T1a   Tumour invades lamina propria or muscularis mucosae

    T1b   Tumour invades submucosa

T2   Tumour invades muscularis propria

T3   Tumour invades adventitia

T4   Tumour invades adjacent structures

    T4a.   Tumour invades pleura, pericardium, azygos vein, diaphragm, or peritoneum

    T4b.   Tumour invades other adjacent structures such as aorta, vertebral body, or trachea

N – Regional Lymph Nodes

NX   Regional lymph nodes cannot be assessed

N0   No regional lymph node metastasis

N1   Metastasis in 1 to 2 regional lymph nodes

N2   Metastasis in 3 to 6 regional lymph nodes

N3   Metastasis in 7 or more regional lymph nodes

M – Distant Metastasis

M0   No distant metastasis

M1   Distant metastasis

pTNM Pathological Classification

The pT and pN categories correspond to the T and N categories. For pM see page 44.

pN0   Histological examination of a regional lymphadenectomy specimen will ordinarily include 7 or more lymph nodes. If the lymph nodes are negative, but the number ordinarily examined is not met, classify as pN0.

Stage and Prognostic Group – Carcinomas of the Oesophagus and Oesophagogastric Junction*

Squamous Cell Carcinoma

Clinical Stage

Stage 0	Tis	N0	M0
Stage I	T1	N0, N1	M0
Stage II	T2	N0, N1	M0
	T3	N0	M0
Stage III	T1, T2	N2	M0
	T3	N1, N2	M0
Stage IVA	T4a, T4b	N0, N1, N2	M0
	Any T	N3	M0
Stage IVB	Any T	Any N	M1

Pathological Stage

Stage	T	N	M
Stage 0	Tis	N0	M0
Stage IA	T1a	N0	M0
Stage IB	T1b	N0	M0
Stage IIA	T2	N0	M0
Stage IIB	T1	N1	M0
	T3	N0	M0
Stage IIIA	T1	N2	M0
	T2	N1	M0
Stage IIIB	T2	N2	M0
	T3	N1, N2	M0
	T4a	N0, N1	M0
Stage IVA	T4a	N2	M0
	T4b	Any N	M0
	Any T	N3	M0
Stage IVB	Any T	Any N	M1

Pathological Prognostic Group

Group	T	N	M	Grade	Location
Group 0	Tis	N0	M0	N/A	Any
Group IA	T1a	N0	M0	1, X	Any
Group IB	T1a	N0	M0	2–3	Any
	T1b	N0	M0	Any	Any
	T2	N0	M0	1	Any
Group IIA	T2	N0	M0	2–3, X	Any
	T3	N0	M0	Any	Lower
	T3	N0	M0	1	Upper, middle
Group IIB	T3	N0	M0	2–3	Upper, middle
	T3	N0	M0	Any	X
	T3	N0	M0	X	Any
	T1	N1	M0	Any	Any
Group IIIA	T1	N2	M0	Any	Any
	T2	N1	M0	Any	Any
Group IIIB	T2	N2	M0	Any	Any
	T3	N1, N2	M0	Any	Any
	T4a	N0, N1	M0	Any	Any
Group IVA	T4a	N2	M0	Any	Any
	T4b	Any N	M0	Any	Any
	Any T	N3	M0	Any	Any
Group IVB	Any T	Any N	M1	Any	Any

Adenocarcinoma

Clinical Stage

Stage 0	Tis	N0	M0
Stage I	T1	N0	M0
Stage IIA	T1	N1	M0
Stage IIB	T2	N0	M0
Stage III	T2	N1	M0
	T3, T4a	N0, N1	M0
Stage IVA	T1–T4a	N2	M0
	T4b	N0, N1, N2	M0
	Any T	N3	M0
Stage IVB	Any T	Any N	M1

Pathological Stage

Stage 0	Tis	N0	M0
Stage IA	T1a	N0	M0
Stage IB	T1b	N0	M0
Stage IIA	T2	N0	M0
Stage IIB	T1	N1	M0
	T3	N0	M0
Stage IIIA	T1	N2	M0
	T2	N1	M0
Stage IIIB	T2	N2	M0
	T3	N1, N2	M0
	T4a	N0, N1	M0
Stage IVA	T4a	N2	M0
	T4b	Any N	M0
	Any T	N3	M0
Stage IVB	Any T	Any N	M1

Pathological Prognostic Group

Group	T	N	M	Grade
Group 0	Tis	N0	M0	N/A
Group IA	T1a	N0	M0	1, X
Group IB	T1a	N0	M0	2
	T1b	N0	M0	1, 2, X
Group IC	T1a, T1b	N0	M0	3
	T2	N0	M0	1, 2
Group IIA	T2	N0	M0	3, X
Group IIB	T1	N1	M0	Any
	T3	N0	M0	Any
Group IIIA	T1	N2	M0	Any
	T2	N1	M0	Any
Group IIIB	T2	N2	M0	Any
	T3	N1, N2	M0	Any
	T4a	N0, N1	M0	Any
Group IVA	T4a	N2	M0	Any
	T4b	Any N	M0	Any
	Any T	N3	M0	Any
Group IVB	Any T	Any N	M1	Any

Note
*The AJCC publishes prognostic groups for adenocarcinoma and squamous cell carcinoma after neoadjuvant therapy (categories with the prefix "y"). See the Executive Editor's Note at the end of this chapter.

Prognostic Factors Grid – Oesophagus

Prognostic factors for survival in oesophageal cancer

Prognostic Factors	Tumour Related	Host Related	Environment Related
Essential	Depth of invasion Lymph node involvement Presence of lymphovascular invasion (LVI)	Performance status Age Nutritional status	Quality of surgery Multimodality approach
Additional	Tumour grading Tumour location	Economic status	Nutritional support
New and promising	CEA, VEGF-C, HER 2		

Source: *UICC Manual of Clinical Oncology*, Ninth Edition. Edited by Brian O'Sullivan, James D. Brierley, Anil K. D'Cruz, Martin F. Fey, Raphael Pollock, Jan B. Vermorken and Shao Hui Huang. © 2015 UICC. Published 2015 by John Wiley & Sons, Ltd.

Editorial Addendum
By Thomas W. Rice, MD, and Eugene H. Blackstone, MD

The 8th editions of the cancer staging manuals for carcinoma of the oesophagus and of the oesophagogastric junction[1,2] are based on modern machine learning analyses of 22,654 patients registered by the Worldwide Esophageal Cancer Collaboration (WECC).[3–8] The Union for International Cancer Control (UICC) definitions vary somewhat from those used to develop the staging recommendations and some categories are undefined by the UICC.

Location (Anatomic Subsites)
The definitions of anatomic subsites (location) used by the UICC differ from that used by the American Joint Committee on Cancer (AJCC) and WECC to develop the staging recommendations. The boundaries used to define the cervical, upper thoracic, middle thoracic and lower thoracic esophagus are defined in Table 1. The AJCC Upper GI Task Force consensus redefined the oesophagogastric junction, such that tumours with epicentres no more than 2 cm into the proximal stomach are staged as oesophageal cancers.

Histologic Grade
Crucial to pathological staging of early squamous cell carcinoma and adenocarcinoma of the oesophagus is the non-anatomic cancer category histologic grade. The definitions suggested for use with these staging recommendations are listed in Tables 2 and 3.

Stage Groups
Analyses of WECC data[6–8] demonstrated the need for separate stage groupings based on AJCC defined classifications

Table 1. Anatomic subsites (location category), defined by the position of the epicentre of the tumour in the oesophagus[1]

Location Category	Definition
X	Location unknown
Cervical	Inferior border of the hypopharynx to sternal notch, 15 cm to 20 cm[#]
Upper	Sternal notch to lower border of azygos vein, >20 cm to 25 cm[#]
Middle	Lower border of azygos vein to lower border of inferior pulmonary veins, >25 cm to 30 cm[#]
Lower	Lower border of inferior pulmonary vein to stomach, including gastroesophageal junction, >30 cm to 40 cm[#]

Typical measurements from the incisor teeth.

Table 2. Histologic grade (G category) for squamous cell carcinoma[*]

G Category	Criteria
G1	Well-differentiated. Prominent keratinization with pearl formation and a minor component of nonkeratinizing basal-like cells. Tumour cells are arranged in sheets, and mitotic counts are low.
G2	Moderately differentiated. Variable histologic features, ranging from parakeratotic to poorly keratinizing lesions. Generally, pearl formation is absent.
G3	Poorly differentiated. Consists predominantly of basal-like cells forming large and small nests with frequent central necrosis. The nests consist of sheets or pavement-like arrangements of tumour cells, and occasionally are punctuated by small numbers of parakeratotic or keratinizing cells. If further testing of "undifferentiated" cancers reveals a squamous cell component, or if after further testing they remain undifferentiated, categorize as squamous cell carcinoma, G3.

Table 3. Histologic grade (G category) for adenocarcinoma[*]

G Category	Criteria
G1	Well differentiated. >95% of tumour is composed of well-formed glands.
G2	Moderately differentiated. 50% to 95% of tumour shows gland formation.
G3	Poorly differentiated. Tumours composed of nest and sheets of cells with <50% of tumour demonstrating glandular formation. If further testing of "undifferentiated" cancers reveals a glandular component, categorize as adenocarcinoma G3.

[*]Reproduced with permission and adapted from Rice TW, Ishwaran H, Ferguson MK, Blackstone EH, Goldstraw P. Cancer of the esophagus and esophagogastric junction: an 8th edition staging primer. *J Thorac Oncol* 2016; in press.[9]

(clinical, pathological, and postneoadjuvant therapy).[1] Additionally separate groupings for histopathologic cell type were required for clinically staged and pathologically staged tumours. UICC adopted *Clinical Stage Groups* in an unaltered state. The UICC listing of *Pathologic Stage Groups* for squamous cell carcinoma and adenocarcinoma without histologic grade and location, which are identical for both histopathologic cell types in this analysis, produced inferior stage grouping of early stage cancers (stage 0–IIB squamous cell carcinoma and stage 0–IIA adenocarcinoma) because of inhomogeneity.[6] Superior pathological grouping with improved homogeneity is afforded by the use of *Pathologic Prognostic Groups* and setting the unknown histologic grade or location to X.

Unique TNM categories (ypTisN1-3M0 and ypT0N0-3M0), dissimilar stage group compositions and markedly different survival profiles compared to clinical and pathological staged patients necessitated separate stage groups, identical for both histopathologic cell types, for those patients who have received neoadjuvant therapy (Postneoadjuvant Therapy). UICC failed to list these groups.

Table 4. Post neoadjuvant therapy stage groups (ypTNM) for squamous cell carcinoma and adenocarcinoma*

Stage	T	N	M
Stage I	T0–2	N0	M0
Stage II	T3	N0	M0
Stage IIIA	T0–2	N1	M0
Stage IIIB	T3	N1	M0
	T0–3	N2	M0
	T4a	N0	M0
Stage IVA	T4a	N1–2	M0
	T4a	NX	M0
	T4b	N0-2	M0
	Any T	N3	M0
Stage IVB	Any T	Any N	M1

*Reproduced with permission and adapted from Rice TW, Ishwaran H, Ferguson MK, Blackstone EH, Goldstraw P. Cancer of the esophagus and esophagogastric junction: an 8th edition staging primer. *J Thorac Oncol* 2016; in press.[9]

References

1. Rice TW, Kelsen D, Blackstone EH, Ishwaran H, Patil DT, Bass AJ, Erasmus JJ, Gerdes H, Hofstetter WL. Esophagus and esophagogastric junction. In: Amin MB, Edge SB, Greene FL, et al., eds. *AJCC Cancer Staging Manual*. 8th ed. New York, NY: Springer; 2017:185-202.
2. Oesophagus including oesophagogastric junction. In: Brierley JD, Gospodarowicz MK, Wittekind C, eds. *TNM Classification of Malignant Tumors. International Union Against Cancer*. 8th ed. Oxford, England: Wiley; 2017:57-62.
3. Rice TW, Apperson-Hansen C, DiPaola LM, et al. Worldwide Esophageal Cancer Collaboration: clinical staging data. *Dis Esophagus*.2016;7:707-14.

4. Rice TW, Lerut TEMR, Orringer MB, et al. Worldwide Esophageal Cancer Collaboration: neoadjuvant pathologic staging data. *Dis Esophagus* 2016;7:715-23.

5. Rice TW, Chen L-Q, Hofstetter WL, et al. Worldwide Esophageal Cancer Collaboration: pathologic staging data. *Dis Esophagus* 2016;7:724-33.

6. Rice TW, Ishwaran H, Hofstetter WL, Kelsen DP, Blackstone EH. Recommendations for pathologic staging (pTNM) of cancer of the esophagus and esophagogastric junction for the 8th edition AJCC/UICC staging manuals. *Dis Esophagus* 2016 (in press).

7. Rice TW, Ishwaran H, Kelsen DP, Hofstetter WL, Blackstone EH. Recommendations for neoadjuvant pathologic staging (ypTNM) of cancer of the esophagus and esophagogastric junction for the 8th edition AJCC/UICC staging manuals. *Dis Esophagus* 2016 (in press).

8. Rice TW, Ishwaran H, Blackstone EH, Hofstetter WL, Kelsen DP. Recommendations for clinical staging (cTNM) of cancer of the esophagus and esophagogastric junction for the 8th edition AJCC/UICC staging manuals. Dis Esophagus 2016 (in press).

9. Rice TW, Ishwaran H, Ferguson MK, Blackstone EH, Goldstraw P. Cancer of the esophagus and esophagogastric junction: an 8th edition staging primer. *J Thorac Oncol* 2016 (in press).

Executive Editor's Note: This chapter has been reprinted from Wittekind Ch, Compton CC, Brierley J, Sobin LH (eds) UICC TNM Supplement A Commentary on Uniform Use, fourth edition, John Wiley & Sons, Ltd., Oxford, 2012. The explanatory notes in this chapter are based on the 7th edition of the TNM classification of carcinoma of the oesophagus and of the oesophagogastric junction. There are important changes in the 8th edition of the classification, mainly in the definition of the oesophagogastric junction, in the classification of regional lymph nodes and in the stages. An Editorial Addendum to this chapter explains the novelties in the 8th edition, but the 7th edition text is included here to facilitate comparison between both editions.

13

Site-Specific Explanatory Notes for Carcinoma of the Oesophagus and of the Oesophagogastric Junction

Rules for Classification

The classification applies to all types of carcinoma. Gastrointestinal stromal tumours and neuroendocrine tumours (carcinoids) have their own classifications. The changes in the 8th edition derive from the analyses of the Worldwide Esophageal Cancer Collaboration (WECC).[1-6]

Oesophagus

Summary – Oesophagus (includes oesophagogastric junction)	
T1	Lamina propria, muscularis mucosae (T1a), submucosa (T1b)
T2	Muscularis propria
T3	Adventitia
T4a	Pleura, pericardium, diaphragm
T4b	Aorta, vertebral body, trachea
N1	1-2 regional
N2	3-6 regional
N3	7 or more regional

A tumour the epicentre of which is in the stomach within 5 cm of the oesophagogastric junction and also extends into the oesophagus is classified and staged using the oesophageal scheme. Tumours with an epicentre in the stomach greater than 5 cm from the oesophagogastric junction or those within 5 cm of the oesophagogastric junction without extension in the oesophagus are classified and staged using gastric carcinoma scheme.

There is a proposal to divide carcinomas of the oesophagogastric junction region into three entities:[7-9]

- Adenocarcinoma of the distal oesophagus (AEG I, so-called Barrett carcinoma)
- 'Real' carcinoma of the cardia (AEG II)
- Subcardial carcinoma of the stomach, infiltrating the distal oesophagus (AEG III)

These proposals give some indication of the epidemiology and biology of the tumours. By sampling worldwide data on oesophageal and oesophagogastric junction cancers, it has been shown that patients with all types of Siewert's carcinoma have a similar poor prognosis to patients with oesophageal cancer.[10,11] Therefore, these different types are classified according to tumours of the oesophagus.

The presence of additional synchronous primary carcinomas that are only histologically demonstrable is classified as multifocality and is not considered in the TNM classificaton. For the separation of these carcinomas from skip metastasis (intramural metastasis), the configuration of tumour cells as well as the presence of intraepithelial neoplasia are considered. In contrast to multi-focality, multiplicity, i.e. the presence of additional macroscopically detectable synchronous primary carcinomas is indicated in brackets, e.g. T2(m) or pT2(3).

So-called skip metastasis (intramural metastasis) are tumour foci (orally or abo-rally) separate from the primary carcinoma in the wall of the oesophagus or stomach particularly in the submucosa. Such skip metastasis can be found in 10-15% in oesophageal tumour resection specimen. They are considered the result of lymphatic spread in the oesophageal wall. These 'skip metastasis' are not considered in the TNM/pTNM classification and are not considered metastasis.

Invasion of adventitia (cT3/pT3) corresponds to invasion of perioesophageal soft tissue. This is not considered invasion of the mediastinum or invasion of adjacent structures (T4).

Invasion of pleura, percardium or diaphragm (structures that are usually considered resectable) are classified as T4a.

A carcinoma of the oesophagus that has invaded the stomach and shows a perforation there is classified as pT4a (equivalent to tumours of the stomach). Invasion of bronchi, lung, heart, aorta, V. cava, V. azygos and invasion of recurrent nerve(s) or phrenic or sympathetic nerves (structures that are usually considered unresectable) are classified as T4b.

Invasion in fistulas between oesophagus and trachea or oesophagus and bronchus or compression of V. cava or V. azygos is classified T4b.

Lymph Nodes (Oesophagus)

The definition of the regional lymph nodes of the oesophagus has been simplified in the 7th edition.

The regional lymph nodes, irrespective of the site of the primary tumour, are those in the oesophageal drainage area including coeliac axis nodes and paraoesophageal nodes in the neck.

Paraoesophageal lymph nodes within the neck are considered regional. All other involved lymph nodes above the clavicles (supraclavicular) are classified as distant metastasis.

In the AJCC Cancer Staging Manual 2009 the regional lymph nodes are listed in detail:

Regional Lymph Nodes

Zone	Number	Site
Supraclavicular	1	Supraclavicular
Upper	2 3p 4 (R, L)	Upper paratracheal Posterior mediastinal/upper paraoesophageal Lower paratracheal (right, left)
AP (aortopulmonary)	5 6	Subaortic aortopulmonary Anterior mediastinal (anterior to ascending aorta ascendens or innominate artery)
Subcarinal	7	Subcarinal
Lower	8 (L,R) 9 (L, R)	Middle paraoesophageal (left, right) Pulmonary ligament (left, right)
Hilar	10 (R, L)	Tracheobronchial (hilar) (right, left)
Thoracal	15	Diaphragmatic
Abdominal	16	Paracardial
	17	Along arteria gastric sinistra
	18	Along arteria hepatica communis
	19	Along arteria lienalis
	20	At the basis of arteria coeliaca

There is a difference in classification of supraclavicular lymph nodes: they are considered as regional in the AJCC Manual, but not in the UICC booklet, where they are designated as distant metastasis.

Another problem arises by the general rule of the TNM system if a tumour involves more than one site or subsite, e.g. contiguous extension to another site or subsite, the regional lymph nodes include those of all involved sites and subsites.

According to this rule, all nodes regional for the stomach have to be considered as regional for tumours of the oesophagus and oesophagogastric junction, too. However, in the AJCC list the following stations are missing: perigastric/lesser curvature, perigastric/greater curvature, suprapyloric, infrapyloric, at the splenic hilum.

Stage Grouping and Prognostic Grouping

The T, N and M categories used by the UICC and the AJCC are identical. The UICC presents two options for stage groupings:

1) A purely anatomical approach that applies to all histological types, and

2) A prognostic AJCC approach that has two separate classifications for squamous cell and adenocarcinoma, with the former taking histological grade and subsite into consideration and the latter including histological grade only. The definitions of the prognostic grouping for squamous cell and adenocarcinoma of UICC and AJCC are identical. The AJCC Manual has only the prognostic scheme.

See Chapter 12 for stage grouping and prognostic groups tables.

References

1. Rice TW, Apperson-Hansen C, DiPaola C et al. Worldwide Esophageal Cancer Collaboration: clinical staging data. *Dis Esophagus* 2016;7: 707-14.

2. Rice TW, Chen L-Q, Hofstetter WL et al. Worldwide Esophageal Cancer Collaboration: pathologic staging data. *Dis Esophagus* 2016;7: 724-33.

3. Rice TW, Lerut TEMR, Orringer MB et al. Worldwide Esophageal Cancer Collaboration: neoadjuvant pathologic staging data. *Dis Esophagus* 2016;7: 715-23.

4. Rice TW, Ishwaran H, Hofstetter WL, Kelsen DP, Blackstone EH. Recommendations for pathologicstaging (pTNM) of cancer of the

esophagus and esophagogastric junction for the 8th edition AJCC/UICC staging manuals. *Dis Esophagus* 2016 (in press).

5. Rice TW, Ishwaran H, Kelsen DP, Hofstetter WL, Blackstone EH. Recommendations for neoadjuvant pathologic staging (ypTNM) of cancer of the esophagus and esophagogastric junction for the 8th edition AJCC/UICC staging manuals. *Dis Esophagus* 2016 (in press).

6. Rice TW, Ishwaran H, Blackstone EH, Hofstetter WL, Kelsen DP. Recommendations for clinical staging (cTNM) of cancer of the esophagus and esophagogastric junction for the 8th edition AJCC/UICC staging manuals. *Dis Esophagus* 2016 (in press).

7. Hermanek P, Henson DE, Hutter RVP, Sobin LH, eds. UICC TNM Supplement 1993. A Commentary on Uniform Use, 1st ed. New York, Wiley; 1993.

8. Sobin LH, Wittekind Ch, eds. UICC TNM Classification of Malignant Tumours, 6th ed. New York, Wiley; 2002.

9. Wittekind Ch, Henson DE, Hutter RVP, Sobin LH, eds. UICC TNM Supplement. A Commentary on Uniform Use, 3rd ed, New York, Wiley; 2003.

10. Rosenberg P, Friederichs J, Schuster T et al. Prognosis of patients with colorectal cancer is associated with lymph node ratio. A single-center analysis of 3026 patients over a 25-year time period. *Ann Surg* 2008; 248: 968-978.

11. Derwinger K, Carlsson G, Gistavsson B. Stage migration in colorectal cancer related to improved lymph node assessment. *Eur J Surg Oncol* 2007; 33: 849-853.

Editorial Addendum

By Thomas W. Rice, MD, and Eugene H. Blackstone, MD

This reprinted manuscript, published in 2012, references material from the UICC 7th edition staging manual. Although some of the material is pertinent today, there are many important changes in the 8th edition.

The Oesophagogastric Junction

The oesophagogastric junction (OGJ) has been redefined for the 8th edition. Use of a simple measurement to define whether a cancer is oesophageal or gastric has impeded OGJ cancer staging since the 1980's. Conflicting statistical analyses necessitated a "place card" consensus decision for the 8th edition. Cancers involving the OGJ that have their epicenter within the proximal 2 cm of the cardia are to be staged as oesophageal cancers. Cancers whose epicenter is more than 2 cm distal from the OGJ, even if the OGJ is involved, will be staged using the stomach cancer TNM and stage groupings.[1] Early work suggests genetic signature of OGJ cancers will be much more useful in appropriate cancer staging by identifying cell of origin rather than relying on gross location.[2,3] A "genetic" definition of the OGJ will obviate the need for further dividing it into thirds (AEG I-III, Siewert I–III). This redefinition of the OGJ will be a focus of the 9th edition staging.

Regional Lymph Nodes

The regional lymph node map has been refined in the 8th edition AJCC staging manual (Figure 22.2).[1] The regional lymph node stations are listed in Table 1. Supraclavicular, perigastric/greater curvature, suprapyloric, infrapyloric, and splenic hilum lymph nodes are non regional lymph nodes in the AJCC 8th edition Cancer Staging Manual.

Stage Grouping and Prognostic Grouping

The recent (7th edition) separation of pathologic groupings into *Pathological Stage* and *Pathological Prognostic Group* by the UICC contradicts the stated purposes of TNM classifications and stage groupings originally set out by the UICC, "Classification is a means of recording facts observed by the clinician whereas staging implies interpretation of these facts regarding prognosis."[4] This superfluous distinction unnecessarily produces confusion and inferior stage grouping (see Chapter 20 Editorial Addendum). With publication of the AJCC 8th edition Cancer Staging Manual and the data-driven placement of oesophageal and OGJ cancers with unknown histologic grade or location the statement "the AJCC manual has only the prognostic scheme" is irrelevant.

References

1. Rice TW, Kelsen D, Blackstone EH, Ishwaran H, Patil DT, Bass AJ, Erasmus JJ, Gerdes H, Hofstetter. Esophagus and esophagogastric junction. In: Amin MB, Edge SB, Greene FL, et al. (Eds.) *AJCC Cancer Staging Manual*. 8th Ed. New York:Springer; 2017:185-202.

2. Cancer Genome Atlas Research Network. Comprehensive molecular characterization of gastric adenocarcinoma. *Nature*. 2014 Sep 11;513:202-9.

3. Hayakawa Y, Sethi N, Sepulveda AR, Bass AJ, Wang TC. Oesophageal adenocarcinoma and gastric cancer: should we mind the gap? *Nat Rev Cancer*. 2016 Apr 26;16:305-18.

4. International Union Against Cancer (UICC). *TNM Classification of Malignant Tumors*. Geneva; 1968.

Table 1. Regional lymph node stations for staging cancer of the oesophagus and oesophagogastric junction

Lymph Node Station	Name	Location
1R	Right lower cervical paratracheal nodes	Between supraclavicular paratracheal space and apex of lung
1L	Left lower cervical paratracheal nodes	Between supraclavicular paratracheal space and apex of lung
2R	Right upper paratracheal nodes	Between intersection of caudal margin of brachiocephalic artery with trachea and apex of lung
2L	Left upper paratracheal nodes	Between top of aortic arch and apex of lung
4R	Right lower paratracheal nodes	Between intersection of caudal margin of brachiocephalic artery with trachea and cephalic border of azygos vein
4L	Left lower paratracheal nodes	Between top of aortic arch and carina
7	Subcarinal nodes	Caudal to carina of trachea
8U	Upper thoracic paraesophageal lymph nodes	From apex of lung to tracheal bifurcation
8M	Middle thoracic paraesophageal lymph nodes	From tracheal bifurcation to caudal margin of inferior pulmonary vein
8Lo	Lower thoracic paraesophageal lymph nodes	From caudal margin of inferior pulmonary vein to oesophagogastric junction
9R	Pulmonary ligament nodes	Within right inferior pulmonary ligament
9L	Pulmonary ligament nodes	Within left inferior pulmonary ligament

continued on next page

15	Diaphragmatic nodes	On dome of diaphragm and adjacent to or behind its crura
16	Paracardial nodes	Immediately adjacent to gastro-esophageal junction
17	Left gastric nodes	Along course of left gastric artery
18	Common hepatic nodes	Immediately on proximal common hepatic artery
19	Splenic nodes	Immediately on proximal splenic artery
20	Celiac nodes	At base of celiac artery

Note: Cervical periesophageal level VI and level VII lymph nodes are named as per the head and neck map.

14

Atlas of Oesophagus and of Oesophagogastric Junction Cancer Staging

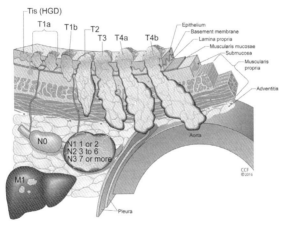

Figure 14.1. Eighth edition TNM categories. T is categorized as Tis: high-grade dysplasia; T1: cancer invades lamina propria, muscularis mucosae, or submucosa and is subcategorized into T1a (cancer invades lamina propria or muscularis mucosae) and T1b (cancer invades submucosa); T2: cancer invades muscularis propria; T3: cancer invades adventitia; T4: cancer invades local structures and is subcategorized as T4a: cancer invades adjacent structures such as pleura, pericardium, azygos vein, diaphragm, or peritoneum and T4b: cancer invades major adjacent structures, such as aorta, vertebral body, or trachea. N is categorized as N0: no regional lymph node metastasis; N1: regional lymph node metastases involving 1 to 2 nodes; N2: regional lymph node metastases involving 3 to 6 nodes; and N3: regional lymph node metastases involving 7 or more nodes. M is categorized as M0: no distant metastasis; and M1: distant metastasis. Copyright ©2016 Cleveland Clinic Foundation, courtesy of Thomas W. Rice, MD.

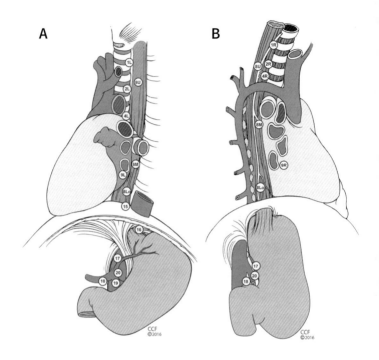

Figure 14.2. Lymph node maps for oesophageal cancer. Regional lymph node stations for staging oesophageal cancer from left **A)**, right **B)**, and anterior **C)**. 1R: Right lower cervical paratracheal nodes, between the supraclavicular paratracheal space and apex of the lung. 1L: Left lower cervical paratracheal nodes, between the supraclavicular paratracheal space and apex of the lung. 2R: Right upper paratracheal nodes, between the intersection of the caudal margin of the brachiocephalic artery with the trachea and apex of the lung. 2L: Left upper paratracheal nodes, between the top of the aortic arch and apex of the lung. 4R: Right lower paratracheal nodes, between the intersection of the caudal margin of the brachiocephalic artery with the trachea and cephalic border of the azygos vein. 4L: Left lower paratracheal nodes, between the top of the aortic arch and the carina. 7: Subcarinal nodes, caudal to the carina of the trachea. 8U: Upper thoracic paraoesophageal lymph nodes, from the apex of the lung to the tracheal bifurcation. 8M: Middle thoracic

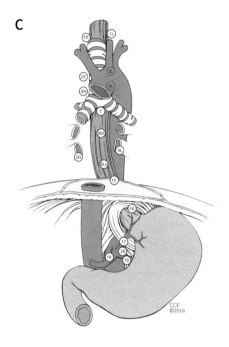

paraoesophageal lymph nodes, from the tracheal bifurcation to the caudal margin of the inferior pulmonary vein. 8Lo: Lower thoracic paraoesophageal lymph nodes, from the caudal margin of the inferior pulmonary vein to the esophagogastric junction. 9R: Pulmonary ligament nodes, within the right inferior pulmonary ligament. 9L: Pulmonary ligament nodes, within the left inferior pulmonary ligament. 15: Diaphragmatic nodes, lying on the dome of the diaphragm and adjacent to or behind its crura. 16: Paracardial nodes, immediately adjacent to the gastrooesophageal junction. 17: Left gastric nodes, along the course of the left gastric artery. 18: Common hepatic nodes, immediately on the proximal common hepatic artery. 19: Splenic nodes, immediately on the proximal splenic artery. 20: Celiac nodes, at the base of the celiac artery. Cervical perioesophageal level VI and level VII lymph nodes are named as per the head and neck map. Copyright ©2016 Cleveland Clinic Foundation, courtesy of Thomas W. Rice, MD.

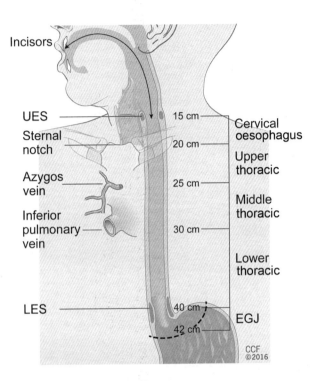

Figure 14.3. Location of oesophageal cancer primary site, including typical endoscopic measurements of each region measured from the incisors. Exact measurements depend on body size and height. Location of cancer primary site is defined by cancer epicenter. Cancers involving the oesophagogastric junction (EGJ) that have their epicenter within the proximal 2 cm of the cardia (Siewert types I/II) are to be staged as oesophageal cancers. Cancers whose epicenter is more than 2 cm distal from the EGJ, even if the EGJ is involved, will be staged using the stomach cancer TNM and stage groups. Key: LES, lower oesophageal sphincter; UES, upper oesophageal sphincter. Copyright ©2016 Cleveland Clinic Foundation, courtesy of Thomas W. Rice, MD.

Index